Rocky, Solid

Dr.Paul Mason on low carb:
Reversing diabetes, losing weight, fiber & lectins

His best obesity and keto diet talks.

Including insulin, autoimmune issues, the gut microbiome and general health

<u>Revised transcripts of his Youtube-Videos</u>

25% of the royalties will be donated to
Dr. Thomas Seyfried's Cancer research!
See www.KetoforCancer.net

Any review would be greatly appreciated to get the message of Dr. Paul Mason out to the public!

TABLE OF CONTENTS

Chapter 1
Evidence based keto: How to lose weight and reverse diabetes

Good morning I'm Dr. Paul Mason and I'm a sports- and exercise medicine physician from Sydney.

Today, we're going to explore the science of ketogenic diets and address the myth, that low-fat diets are good for weight loss. We're going to learn how to reverse the supposedly irreversible type 2 diabetes, and discover exactly what it is about vegetable oils that makes them toxic.

I'd like to start by introducing cognitive psychologist Dr. T. This is Dr. T:

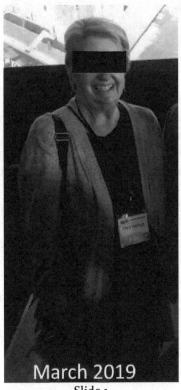

March 2019

Slide 1

Now, who here thinks she looks lazy or greedy? Of course, this is a ridiculous question, you can't possibly tell just by looking at her. And yet, that is a conclusion that many people would come to when they looked at an old photo of her:

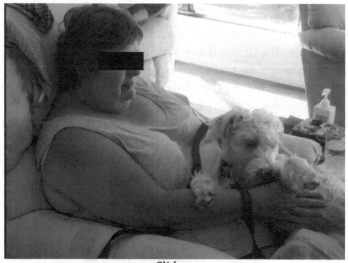

Slide 2

This is because we've been indoctrinated that obesity is a conscious decision, that choosing to be greedy and lazy is the sole reason that most people become obese.

Now, it's not exactly as if Dr. T wasn't motivated to lose weight. It was having a massive impact on the quality of her life:

"It was miserable, every day. I can't remember a day I didn't wake up and think *I'll just start the diet on Monday,* or *If I could just fix my weight problem, I could get my life together!"*

Clearly, she also wasn't overweight because she didn't exercise:

"Well, I always rode to and from work, which was about 25 to 30 km roundtrip. We would plan holidays that were cycling holidays. I would walk... I had a dog, I would walk my dog for an hour in the afternoon.

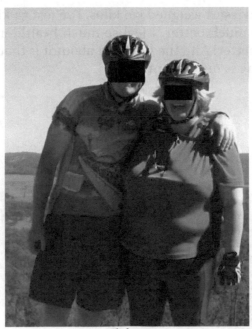

Slide 3

I would go to the gym, I signed up with weight management clinics at the University I worked with, where I worked with exercise physiology students and dieticians. So I would be going - and I was the one who always showed up! I never missed a session. I was there all the time! And then, I would go on the days I didn't have to go."

And nor was she overweight because she didn't follow medical advice:

"I've tried all the diets! I've tried the eating plans, I've tried drugs: I tried Xenical - my doctor, at one stage, wanted to put me on amphetamines... but I kind of value my brain a bit too much for that.

And by my 40s, things were so out of control that I actually tried bariatric surgery! I went in and had a lap band. Because I honestly thought:

The worst case, I won't get any fatter - and the best case, by some miracle, I may actually get back to a normal size."

And even that failed! Despite all of these failed attempts, Dr. T eventually found a way to succeed and got her life back:

"At my heaviest, I weighed 130 kilos. I've lost 55 kilos to date! My life is so much better, I feel so much healthier - every aspect of it is better! And the best part about it is that I don't feel like my eating is out of control."

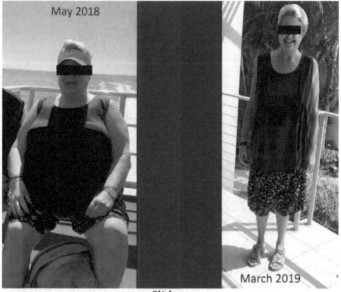

May 2018

March 2019

Slide 4

So the question is: What did she do? Well, clearly it wasn't following the conventional medical wisdom - because following this advice had only led her to get fatter and sicker. No.

Her breakthrough came when she understood that obesity is not so much about calories as it is about insulin. Let's take a look at the evidence that insulin, a hormone secreted into our blood, can make us fat:

This is a picture of a 34 year old female who had an insulinoma, a tumor producing insulin. In this picture, she's 107 kilograms and she's only 152 centimeters tall. And then, she had surgery to remove the tumor.

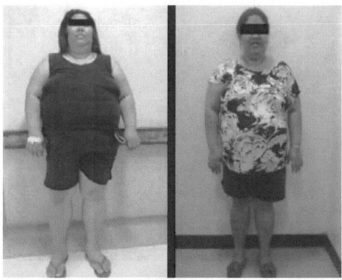

Slide 5

This stopped the excess insulin production.. and over the next 50 days, she lost 18 kilograms, without any change in diet or exercise! Just reduced insulin levels!

And anyone who's ever had to inject insulin understands that it simulates fat storage. Continued injection of insulin into the same site, over a period of time, often leads to a condition called lipohypertrophy - quite literally *fat enlargement.* This manifests as a localized accumulation of fat tissue at different insulin injection sites - and about a quarter of every type 1 diabetic patient will develop this.

Furthermore, high insulin levels in the blood is highly predictive of future weight gain. This study followed initially lean subjects for 8 years, to see who developed obesity. Those who were in the lowest 25% for their insulin levels, at the start and end of the eight-year period, had only a 2% chance of becoming obese.

What about those in the highest 25%? They had a risk of becoming obese of over 70%! And on average, they were 50% heavier:

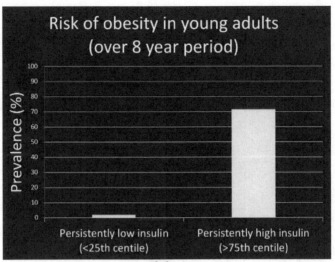
Slide 6

So if high insulin levels plays an important role in obesity, it's only logical to ask: What raises insulin levels? And the answer is found in our diet! Or more precisely, the carbohydrate content of our diet.

When we eat fat, we only get a small rise in insulin levels. We get somewhat of a larger response of protein - which is actually a good thing, because insulin helps build our lean tissues, like muscle. But it's when we get to carbohydrates that the story starts getting really interesting:

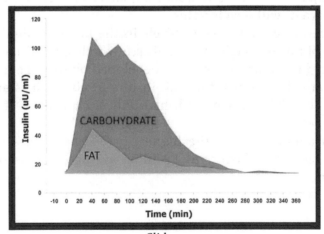
Slide 7

When we directly compare the insulin release by carbohydrates and fat, we understand why carbohydrates are fattening and fat itself is not.

And one of the reasons why insulin levels impact our weight gain is that (amongst other things) it helps regulate our involuntary energy expenditure, even at rest. This was elegantly shown in this recent study, where subjects were allocated to either a low 20%, moderate 40% or a high 60% carbohydrate diet.

Then, the investigators did something really interesting: They adjusted the energy intake of the subjects to prevent any weight change. What they found was that the low carbohydrate group, in blue (left side), actually had an increased energy expenditure!

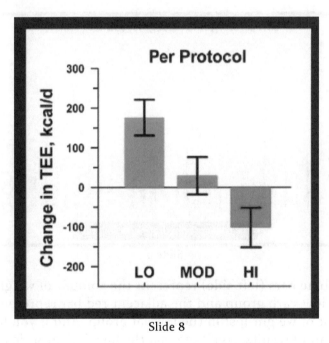

Slide 8

And this compared to the high carbohydrate group in red (right), which had a reduced energy expenditure.

The difference between these two groups was very significant, about 278 kilocalories a day. This is basically equivalent to the amount of energy expended in one hour of moderate intensity exercise. In fact, 278 kilocalories a day would

9

translate into a 10 kilogram weight loss over 3 years in a 30 year old man.

And this is not an isolated finding: In fact, amongst high-quality randomized controlled trials, you could even say there's a consensus. Using the definitions of **low-carb** as

- less than 130 grams a day, and
- low-fat as less than 35% energy,

let's have a look at the available evidence.

So between 2003 and 2018, there were 62 randomized controlled trials that compared weight loss on either a low-carb or a low-fat diet. Of these 62 studies, 31 of them did not find statistically significant results - which means 31 did!

Here, I've graphed the results of all of these studies:

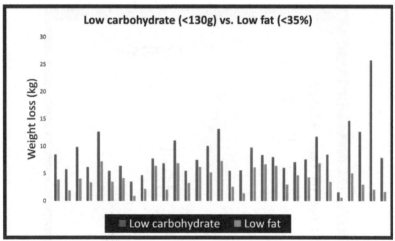

Slide 9

The blue bars (left side) represent the amount of weight lost in the low-carb group and the adjacent red bar represents the amount of weight lost in the low-fat group. And if you look at each pair of results, you'll see that the low-carb arms lost more weight... in all of them. All of them! Not one single study with statistically significant results was found in favor of low-fat diets for weight loss!

So if you were wanting to lose weight, which diet would you choose?

Now, let's take a closer look at carbohydrates. Most of us instinctively know that sugar can be bad for us. But did you realize that carbohydrates are literally made of sugar? Just a string of glucose molecules?

Even complex carbs such as brown rice and sweet potato contain this glucose. And when we digest these carbs, each and every one of these glucose molecules will end up in our bloodstream.

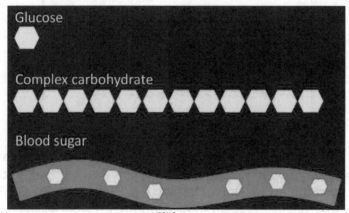

Slide 10

Now, this may not necessarily pose a problem. First of all, we can actually metabolize or burn some of the glucose - and we can also store some in our muscle and liver as glycogen. In fact, healthy people can store about 80% percent of the glucose as glycogen.

But this all changes if we have too much carbohydrates. In this study, subjects were deliberately fed too much carbohydrate, just to see what would happen. Well, some of the carbohydrate was oxidized or burnt as you can see in the blue bars: (CHO oxidation)

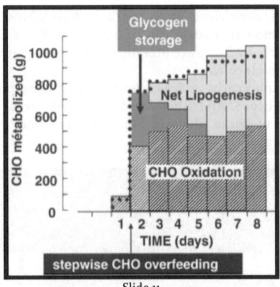
Slide 11

But this was relatively constant, right through the duration of the study, right through to day 8. Meaning, that putting more carbohydrates into the system did not increase how much was burnt! And some of the glucose that wasn't burnt was stored as glycogen, as we've already seen.

But this capacity was reduced over the few subsequent days, as the stores progressively filled up. Until by day 6, there was no spare storage capacity at all. What then happened with the leftover carbohydrate? Well, that was turned into fat - via this process called de novo lipogenesis!

And as the storage capacity continued to reduce, this fat production continued to increase. The fat that was produced is called a triglyceride fat. This triglyceride can be then carried around in our circulation.

So now we have a trifecta, three things from eating carbs:
- Increased blood glucose levels
- Increased insulin levels, and
- Circulating triglycerides.

And these are three key ingredients for the storage of fat.

So each and every fat cell in the body is in contact with blood vessels and that exposes them to these circulating factors, the glucose, the insulin, the triglycerides. Let's see what happens, let's look at triglycerides first:

In its complete form, it's unable to enter the fat cell. This is where insulin comes in: Insulin stimulates this enzyme here, lipoprotein lipase, which then cleaves the larger molecule and allows these fatty acids to then diffuse across into the fat cell.

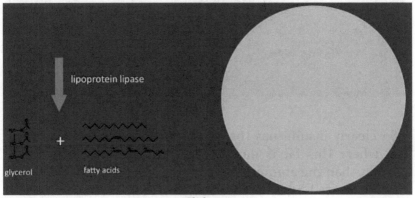

Slide 12

Insulin also activates this glut 4 transporter which is like a gate that allows glucose to enter the fat cell. And once inside the fat cell, the glucose is converted into glycerol. This then combines with the fatty acids to reform a triglyceride - and this is how fat is stored under the influence of insulin.

But if you want to lose weight, then the triglyceride must be sliced up again to allow to exit the fat cell for metabolism - and this requires activity of an enzyme called hormone sensitive lipase. This separates the glycerol from the fatty acids, allowing them to leave the fat cell.

Insulin blocks this enzyme, puts the brakes on it! And without this step, the fat can't be metabolized. Insulin blocks fat burning!

So putting it all together, we can see that insulin pushes fatty acids and glucose into fat cells... and then for extra insult, it prevents them from leaving. A triple whammy!

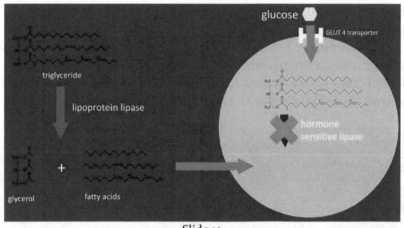

Slide 13

So clearly insulin has the capacity to stimulate fat storage. But where this fat is deposited is probably even more important than the amount of fat.

Shown in red here (inner area) is what is known as visceral fat. In and around the organs. And it's this pattern of fat deposition that is most strongly associated with liver disease and type 1 diabetes.

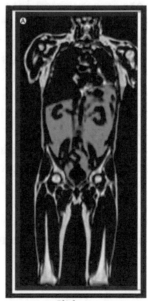

Slide 14

In fact, for every one kilogram increase in visceral fat the risk of diabetes in males is doubled - and for females quadrupled! Process that for a second. As a female, if you were to have one extra kilogram of visceral fat, your risk of diabetes would be increased by 4 times! And this is because fatty liver disease directly contributes to something called insulin resistance, which is at the heart of type 2 diabetes.

Now, it's worth focusing for a moment on just what exactly insulin resistance means. It refers to our tissues being resistant to the effects of insulin. In other words, the insulin that we have just doesn't work as well - and to compensate, our pancreas releases more.

So insulin resistance can often be identified by the high levels of insulin that result from this compensatory response. Now, we know that insulin is able to stimulate the storage of glucose in muscle and liver, as glycogen. But in the case of insulin resistance, this storage is impaired and we end up with higher levels of glucose in the circulation. And this excess blood glucose can be turned into fat through the process of de novo lipogenesis.

On the left side here, we see the degree of de novo lipogenesis following a high carbohydrate meal in healthy subjects, without insulin resistance.

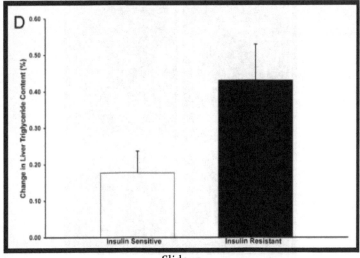

Slide 15

And the response for the same meal in insulin resistant subjects is more than doubled! This is a direct consequence of the insulin resistance associated with fatty liver.

Fortunately, visceral fat and fatty liver is extremely sensitive to weight loss on a low carbohydrate diet. This is a DEXA-scan of one of my patients and you can see the visceral fat concentrated around the region of the liver.

Now after going on a low-carb diet, and losing only 9% body weight, you can see a big reduction in the visceral fat stores. And this effect is even seen on low-carb diets... even, when we deliberately overfeed to prevent weight loss, we get this redistribution of fat.

We also see it with exercise. While it doesn't reliably lead to weight loss, it certainly leads to this redistribution of fat. And that's how we're beginning to understand why some people can be metabolically healthy and still be overweight!

Of course, the reverse is also true: It's possible to be skinny and metabolically unwell. That is a person we call TOFI: Thin on the outside, fat on the inside.

And this is clearly demonstrated on these DEXA scans: The man on the left has a BMI of only 25 - and yet he's got masses of visceral fat. The man on the right has a BMI of 30, technically obese.

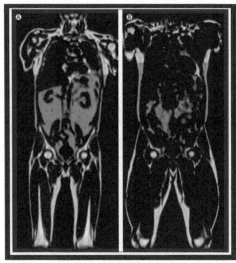

Slide 16

And yet he's only got one-third of the amount of visceral fat. And this only serves to illustrate the limitations of using BMI to assess metabolic health.

Much more accurate and very simple is to simply take measure around the waist, abdominal circumference. This better reflects visceral mass.

There's also other signs, other external signs of insulin resistance we can have a look at. Let's hear from Dr. T again:

"And everybody I speak to has no idea that skin tags are a pretty good indicator of insulin resistance. They all go *Oh really?*"

Unfortunately, this is not common knowledge. I've lost count at the number of patients who come in with skin tags who tell me the story that their doctor doesn't know what causes them... but is still very, very keen to burn them off.

We can also see this characteristic pattern of skin pigmentation, usually in the armpits, from the groin. Sometimes it's on the back of the fingers, around the neck.

Acne is also associated with insulin resistance, and this is a major benefit that many of my younger patients often report. There's also laboratory testing we can do for insulin resistance. In my clinic, I measure both glucose and insulin levels over two hours after giving them a drink of glucose, 75 grams.

This allows me to grade the severity of insulin resistance. And it falls on a continuum, from very mild insulin resistance - without a rise in blood sugar - all the way up to full-blown, insulin dependent, type 2 diabetes.

So let's look at the standard testing for diabetes: That only looks at glucose levels. And the problem with only looking at glucose levels is that even with the onset of insulin resistance, the compensatory increase in insulin levels usually keeps glucose levels within the normal range for quite some time!

This graph is an example of glucose levels in a typical diabetic patient in the years leading up to their diagnosis:

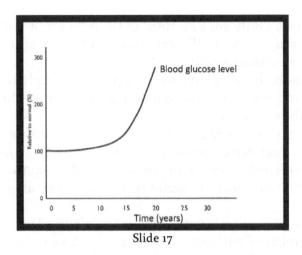

Slide 17

You can see that the glucose doesn't really rise until about 10 years... at which point, pre-diabetes may finally be diagnosed. What happens if we look at insulin levels over the same period of time? We can detect the problem much earlier!

Here we see that progressive increase in insulin levels which occurs in response to the resistance:

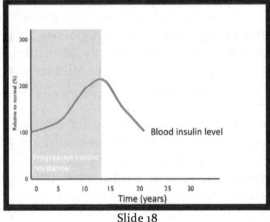

Slide 18

This most commonly occurs as a result of excess carbohydrate. Then, as the pancreas (which secretes the insulin) begins to fail, insulin some levels fall.

Let's now look at glucose and insulin levels together: This vertical dash line represents a state where both glucose and insulin levels are normal. And over time, with the onset of insulin resistance, insulin levels rise - but blood sugar is still normal! So on a standard blood test only looking at glucose, everything still looks hunky-dory. Not even pre-diabetic!

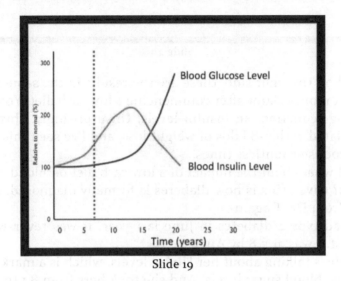

Slide 19

But looking at the insulin level we can begin to see a problem. Finally, the increase in insulin levels can't completely compensate for the insulin resistance - and blood glucose levels begin to rise! This is when pre-diabetes is conventionally diagnosed, often a decade or more after insulin resistance has began to occur.

All the while, the patient has probably been suffering the effects of high insulin levels, such as weight gain and increasing blood pressure.

Then, as the cells in the pancreas begin to fail, insulin secretion falls. And the combined state of reduced insulin levels and insulin resistance often leads to a precipitous rise in blood sugar levels - and this is where diabetes is diagnosed. Possibly two decades after it all began!

Fortunately, this process is reversible on a low-carb diet. On the left, these are the insulin results of one of my patients on one of these two hour tests.

	February 2016		August 2016	
	Insulin		Insulin	
Fasting	8	mU/L	4	mU/L
1 Hour	114	mU/L	71	mU/L
2 Hours	13	mU/L	12	mU/L

Slide 20

And on the right side, these are the results in the same patient six months later after commencing a low carb diet. You can see big reductions in insulin levels. Unsurprisingly, this was associated with 7-8 kilos of weight loss, and I've seen this type of response countless times.

And what about the impact of a low carb diet on blood sugar levels? Given this is how diabetes is formally diagnosed. Let's hear from Dr. T again:

"I had type 2 diabetes in June last year. It was reversed by August, I was at 5.8 by August."

So she's talking about her HbA1c levels, which is a marker of average blood sugar levels. And she took hers from 8.1 to 5.8 - which is an excellent response. And this is consistent with diabetes reversal!

This graph here shows how rapid the improvements can be:

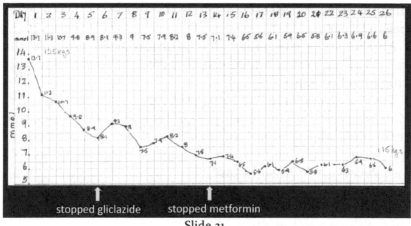

Slide 21

20

This graph was recorded by a 71 year old gentleman, who dropped his morning fasting blood glucose levels quite literally in half - in only two weeks! All the while, he stopped two diabetic medications over the same period.

This study here confirms that the reversal of diabetes is possible on scale. The grey line (upper line) shows the average blood sugar level in patients receiving standard diabetic care over a two-year period:

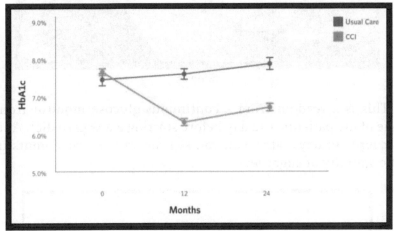

Slide 22

The bottom, light blue line shows the average sugar levels of diabetic patients on a low-carb diet. You can clearly see that those receiving standard diabetic care had significantly higher blood sugar levels over the two-year period. In fact, at 2 years, 53% of the patients on the low-carb diets met the criteria for diabetes reversal!

Now, given that most of the glucose in our circulation comes from what we eat, it's possible to see major improvements quite literally over night, when we start a low carb diet.

This is a continuous glucose monitor sensor. It sits on the back of the upper arm and has a small painless needle which senses glucose levels. It communicates wirelessly with a smartphone or a dedicated reader device, and provides 24-hour realtime blood sugar monitoring.

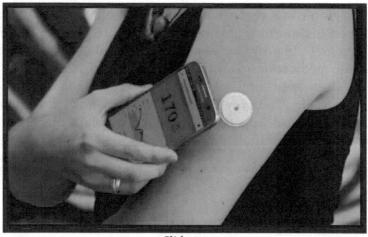

Slide 23

This is a readout from a continuous glucose monitor from one of my patients, the day before starting a low carb diet. And a couple of days later, you can see the vast improvements in the stability of sugar levels:

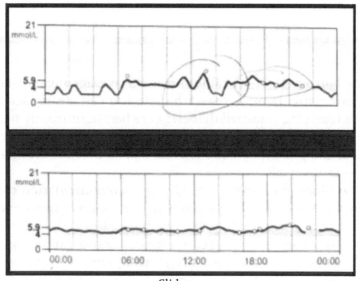

Slide 24

This kind of stability is perhaps even more important than the absolute level. Because it's the variations in the blood sugar levels which generates significant amounts of oxidative stress... which, as we'll soon see, causes problems in and of itself.

I do recommend these monitors to a lot of patients. To anybody, who's curious about their personal blood sugar response to specific foods. It's also a great compliance tool: You can't pretend that something is okay. The evidence there is staring you in the face.

It's what I call real-time accountability. And for many patients, this helps them to stick to a low-carb diet.

I'd like to now shift gears and have a look at processed foods. Processed foods actually now make up more than half of the consumed dietary energy in most westernized countries, high-income countries.

Despite often being disguised behind packaging making various health claims, they're really not that good for us. When I think about processed foods, I think of two key ingredients: Sugar and vegetable oils. Or more correctly seed oils. Let's start with sugar.

Sugar or sucrose is a problem because it contains fructose. Exactly 50 percent in fact, which is very comparable to the amount of fructose in high fructose corn syrup. So we don't get away with it in Australia.

The first problem is that fructose is very sweet, even compared to glucose. Fructose is actually about 2.5 times sweeter than glucose - and this means that fructose is more rewarding to us.

There is a pathway in the brain, the mesolimbic pathway, that is activated by sweet taste. It's a reward pathway, and there's no doubt that a degree of addiction contributes to both cravings and overeating related to this pathway, in the state of obesity.

Almost paradoxically: In obesity, the dopamine receptors are reduced. So you can see on this brain scan, there's less dopamine receptors in the brain of the obese individual than there is in the normal weight individual:

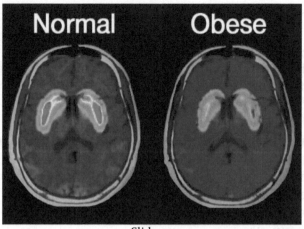

Slide 25

This means that for the same level of reward, an obese person needs to consume either more or sweeter foods - and this is part of the pathway that drives them to things like sugar and fructose. And fructose is involved in both causing this process and continuing this cycle.

Fructose consumption also leads to much more fat production. Remember that de novo lipogenesis? Well, as we know, in a metabolically healthy state most of the glucose can be taken up by the liver and by muscle tissues, and only about 20% will actually contribute to the novo lipogenesis.

Fructose on the other hand has no capacity to be stored! All the fructose you ingest will contribute to fat production via this de novo lipogenesis.

And fructose can be hidden! These are all different names for sugars, most of them containing fructose, that are used in food labeling:

•Agave nectar/syrup	•Evaporated cane juice	•Maltose
•Barley malt	•Fructose	•Maple syrup
•Beet sugar	•Fruit juice	•Molasses
•Blackstrap molasses	•Fruit juice concentrate	•Muscovado
•Brown sugar	•Glucose	•Palm sugar
•Cane sugar	•Golden syrup	•Panela
•Carob syrup	•Grape sugar/syrup	•Powdered sugar
•Caster sugar	•High-fructose corn syrup	•Rapadura
•Coconut sugar	(HFCS)	•Raw sugar
•Coffee sugar crystals	•Honey	•Rice syrup
•Confectioner's sugar	•Icing sugar	•Sucrose
•Corn syrup	•Invert sugar	•Sugar
•Date sugar/syrup	•Lactose	•Treacle
•Demerara	•Malt	•Turbinado
•Dextrose	•Maltodextrin	•White sugar

Slide 26

Take for example a random almond milk, boldly proclaiming that it contains "No cane sugar". But when we look at the ingredients, we may find this: "Organic agave syrup" - and this is actually even worse than sucrose, because it contains 75% fructose! Typical of many processed foods, almond milks also often contain vegetable oil. Why? I don't know.

But this poses a significant issue. It's not solely due to the omega 6 fat content. Vegetable oils are high in linoleic acid, which is an omega 6 fat. And it was assumed by many, including myself, that this linoleic acid would be converted first to arachidonic acid and then to these inflammatory molecules down the bottom, called eicosanoids.

The problem with this line of thinking though is that arachadonic acid is only converted to these inflammatory molecules, if there's an inflammatory trigger of sorts. That is: The production of leukotrienes, thromboxanes and prostaglandins needs an inflammatory stimuli. It requires activation of these enzymes that occur in inflammatory states:

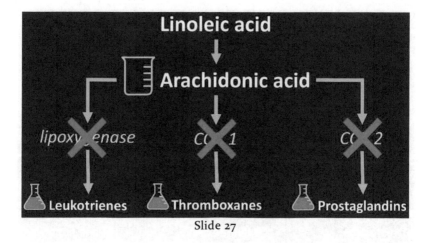
Slide 27

And in a low inflammatory state - such as on a low carbohydrate diet - these enzymes are less active. So a archadonic acid in and of itself is not inherently inflammatory, and it can actually increase in a low inflammatory state.

It's also likely that stabilization of blood glucose levels on a low-carb diet, by reducing the oxidative stress, actually reduces the damage to the arachidonic acid in our cell membranes, also increasing the levels.

And this is exactly what we see. So in this recent study, comparing low carb and high carbohydrate diets, we can see the low-carb intervention actually had significantly higher levels of plasma arachidonic acid than the high carb diet.

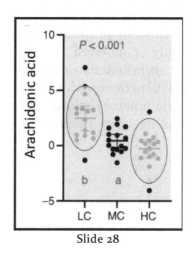
Slide 28

Furthermore, arachidonic acid is essential for good health. It's an essential component of our cell membranes and, among other things, it's involved in muscle repair and growth, and the growth and repair of neurons. So the problem with vegetable oils is not the omega 6 content itself, but the tendency for vegetable oils to become oxidized.

When we have a look at saturated fats, they're quite resistant to oxidation because they lack double bonds between the carbon atoms.

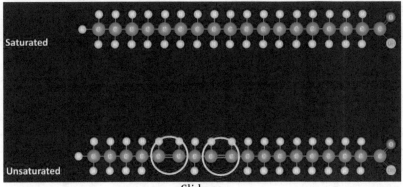

Slide 29

But when we have a look at unsaturated fats, they do have these double bonds which are very reactive and prone to oxidation. And the more double bonds a fat has, the more likely it is to be oxidized.

Here we can see the tendency of fats to oxidize with cooking, ranging from the largely saturated fat lard on the left, through to the polyunsaturated sunflower oil with multiple double bonds on the right:

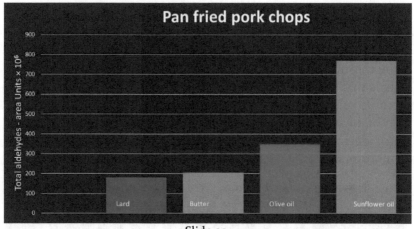
Slide 30

And you can see that olive oil in the third column, with it's single double bond, sits somewhere in the middle.

Even if you don't cook vegetable oils, they're still prone to oxidation. This study measured progressive oxidation in walnut oil stored over eight days:

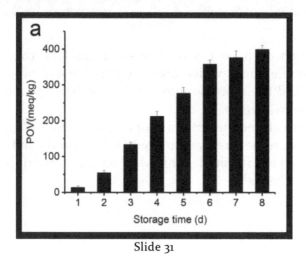
Slide 31

And you can see a massive increase in oxidation products in a matter of days! This is why vegetable oils have antioxidants added to them. Even then, though, the oxidation is only reduced and it's not completely eliminated.

After you ingest oxidized oils, you absorb them. They get absorbed through the small intestine, in particles called chylomicrons. Whereupon they get transported in the circulation to the liver. And this oxidized load to the liver activates an inflammatory response - and ultimately, it contributes to insulin resistance.

And it should be noted that these inflammatory effects are not isolated to the liver, it also occurs in other organs such as the kidneys and the lungs.

This graph here compares the absorption of oxidized fats to these chylomicrons, between a meal containing low oxidation levels and a meal with high oxidized levels:

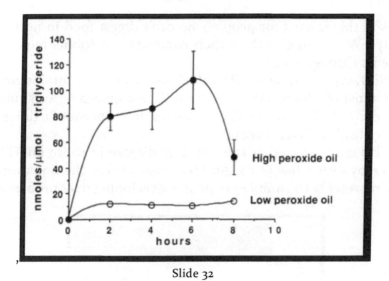

Slide 32

Clearly, we can absorb these oxidation products.

With the help of electron microscope pictures of a mouse liver, we have found how these oxidized fats can accumulate in the liver. This accumulation is associated with a pronounced inflammatory response and the development of fatty liver. This leads to a fibrosis, typical a fatty liver. This condition is almost always immediately adjacent to those oxidized fats.

We also see clear evidence of this in humans. This is TPN, total parenteral nutrition:

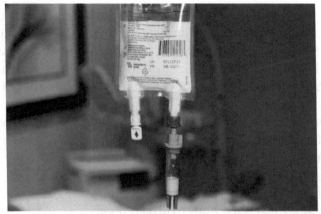

Slide 33

And this is used for people who can't digest food in normal ways. We try to give them their complete nutritional requirements through a vain.

Now, typical of most TPN infusions... this bag contains 20% fat, most of which is the highly oxidizable omega 6. And quite predictably, infusion of TPN - with its rich content of oxidized fats - leads to liver disease!

This study looked at rates of liver disease in those on TPN therapy over a few years. And the amount that the line drops by represents the number of people developing liver problems:

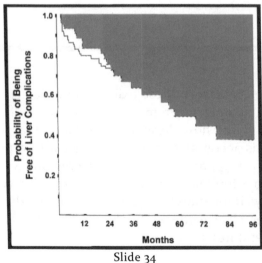

Slide 34

You can see that the percentage of people with biopsy proven liver disease, after 7 years of TPN therapy, was about 60 % - and this trend showed no signs of stopping!

In fact, several patients died of liver disease over the course of this study! So clearly, the ingestion of oxidized vegetable oils is probably not good for the liver.

Do you know what could be worse, though? The consumption of oxidized oils if you're a poorly controlled diabetic. The bar on the left represents the degree of oxidation products absorbed into chylomicrons following a meal of oxidized corn oil. In healthy subjects.

The middle bar: The same meal of oxidized corn oil in well controlled type 2 diabetics - and if you're a poorly controlled type 2 diabetic, then all bets are off, this is represented by the bar on the right side:

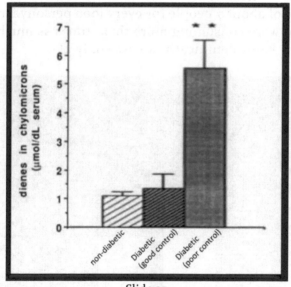

Slide 35

This is why control of blood sugar is so important. If you're a poorly controlled diabetic consuming vegetable oils, you're on a hiding to nothing,

So then, what to do? Well, first of all keep: Your blood sugar level low and get your polyunsaturated fats from fresh food. So long as the food you're eating is not rancid... actually, the

31

definition of rancidity is oxidized fats... you're probably going to be okay.

This doubly applies to omega 3s, which are even more prone to oxidation than Omega 6s. So you've got a choice between supplements - which are probably oxidized - or fresh food.

And you might also want to discuss with your doctor something like melatonin which is a potent antioxidant. And predictably, it's actually been shown in research, to reliably reverse fatty liver disease.

Now, some of you will have heard all of this, and you'll still be uncomfortable with the idea of eating saturated fat. Well, this prospective study looked at more than 150,000 participants and followed them for 7 years and looked at saturated fat consumption and mortality rates.

And it found, that those habitually consuming about 10 percent of their calories from saturated fat (not much), had a death rate of about 7 people for every 1000 personyears. But in those who were consuming more than times as much saturated fat, the equivalent death rate was only 4!

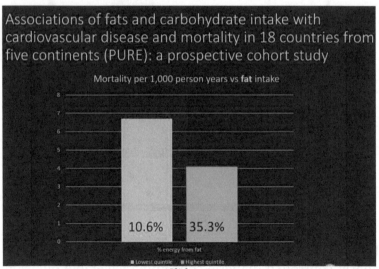

Slide 36

And there was no upper level of saturated fat intake which appeared problematic - as energy from saturated fat increased, so too did the benefits.

Yes, I know that saturated fat can increase LDL cholesterol - and No! That doesn't matter either! This systematic review from 2016 looked at 19 cohort studies with over 68,000 participants:

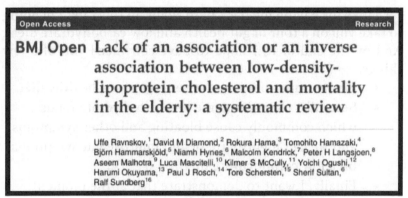

Open Access

Research

BMJ Open Lack of an association or an inverse association between low-density-lipoprotein cholesterol and mortality in the elderly: a systematic review

Uffe Ravnskov,[1] David M Diamond,[2] Rokura Hama,[3] Tomohito Hamazaki,[4] Björn Hammarskjöld,[5] Niamh Hynes,[6] Malcolm Kendrick,[7] Peter H Langsjoen,[8] Aseem Malhotra,[9] Luca Mascitelli,[10] Kilmer S McCully,[11] Yoichi Ogushi,[12] Harumi Okuyama,[13] Paul J Rosch,[14] Tore Schersten,[15] Sherif Sultan,[6] Ralf Sundberg[16]

Slide 37

Of those 19 studies, 16 of them found an inverse relationship between the level of LDL cholesterol and risk of mortality. That is: The higher the LDL level, the lower the risk of dying. And 14 of those studies reached statistical significance, meaning this finding was very unlikely to be due to chance.

So to close: Remember that obesity is treatable and diabetes is reversible. All you have to do is

- limit your carbohydrates, especially sugar
- avoid vegetable oils and
- embrace saturated fat.

A pretty simple recipe. And I'd also like to offer a public thanks to Dr. T who shared her journey, in the hope that it might help others, suffering from the same problems and issues that she did.

If you're a doctor, please be open to the possibility that what you've learnt in medical school may be wrong. And if your patients come to you wanting to try keto, support them! Their lives might depend on it!

Thank you.

Chapter 2
From fibre to the microbiome: Low carb gut health

Thanks for having me back here again. In this talk, I'm going to take you on a tour of gut health and low carbohydrate diets. And by the end of it, I hope to have convinced you of a few things:

- Firstly, that fiber is not a necessity for a healthy diet.
- Secondly, there are some low carbohydrate foods which commonly cause bloating and other symptoms, and we can identify these and improve gut symptoms on a low carbohydrate diet.
- Finally, I want to demonstrate that at the moment there's simply not enough evidence that altering our gut bacteria can lead to weight loss.

So let's start with fiber. This is defined as the carbohydrate portion of plant foods which we can't digest. Remember, fiber only comes from plant foods.

It can be divided into two types: we have a soluble fiber... and this is readily able to be fermented by the bacteria in our colons, and this produces gas and something called short chain fatty-acids.

Then we have insoluble fiber, that's much more resistant to being broken down by the bacteria in our colon. This is the type of fiber that adds bulk to our stools.

Now, there's been a lot of suggested benefits to the ingestion of fiber. This includes preventing bowel cancer, preventing diverticulosis, helping hemorrhoids, lowering blood sugar levels, and, of course, treating constipation.

In fact, it is now conventional wisdom that fiber is a necessary component of a healthy diet. So... understandably, many of my patients are concerned about the potential impacts of removing high carbohydrate cereals and breads from their diet.

In the Australian diet, these represent 45% of the fiber that the average Australian gets. And when we have a look at the

the current governmental advice, they consider that fiber is the best available treatment for constipation, surpassed by none.

But this opinion doesn't bear any scientific scrutiny.

American Journal of Gastroenterology
© 2005 by Am. Coll. of Gastroenterology
Published by Blackwell Publishing

ISSN 0002-9270
doi: 10.1111/j.1572-0241.2004.40885.x

Myths and Misconceptions About Chronic Constipation

Stefan A. Müller-Lissner, M.D., Michael A. Kamm, M.D., F.R.C.P.,
Carmelo Scarpignato, M.D., D.Sc., F.A.C.G., and Arnold Wald, M.D., F.A.C.G.
Park-Klinik Weissensee, Berlin, Germany; St. Marks Hospital, London, UK; Laboratory of Clinical Pharmacology, Department of Human Anatomy, Pharmacology and Forensic Sciences, University of Parma, Parma, Italy; and University of Pittsburgh Medical Center, Pittsburgh, USA

Slide 1

Now, for such a widely accepted and believed claim, you'd think there would be compelling evidence to back it up. Except there's not!

I could not locate one randomized controlled trial, expressly looking at symptoms of constipation. Sure, there's trials looking at bulk- and transit rate and a few other things like that, but when we look at the symptoms of constipation, the research just isn't there.

So, I'd like to present to you the best trial that I could find. This was a case control study. So in this study, 63 patients who presented with constipation were recruited, and high and low fiber diets were compared in these patients.

This also included a zero fiber diet that required the complete cessation of all vegetables, cereals, fruits, wholemeal breads and rice.

This graph here represents the percentage of study participants before the study, suffering from each of the symptoms listed on the right side.

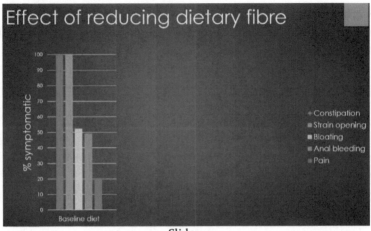

Slide 2

You can see, before the study started, all of them had constipation, and strain opening their bowels - and a number also experienced bloating, bleeding, and pain.

When the study participants... those who went on a high-fiber diet, we can see that the proportion and suffering symptoms actually increased, especially bloating.

Then there was a reduced fiber arm, and what you can see here is that those on the reduced fiber diet actually demonstrated a modest reduction in symptoms.

So, the question is: What happened to those, the majority of those in the study, who had zero fiber in their diet?

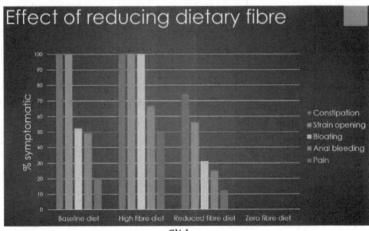

Slide 3

This is not a mistake! (Far right side, no bars at all) I didn't just forget to put something in the slide there. Not one patient on the zero fiber diet had any symptoms! That's quite astonishing, really - and these findings were highly statistically significant. Highly. They weren't due to random chance.

Now, just out of interest: Every single person in the zero fiber group, ended up having one bowel action per day, every day. How did this compare to those in the high-fiber group? One bowel action on average every 6.83 days. Still think that fiber is good for constipation?

To understand why fiber reduces constipation, gives such striking results, let's look at the diagnostic criteria that we as doctors use to diagnose functional constipation. And you'll note that each one of these criterion relates to ease of passage of stool through the anal sphincter. Which is quite logical, really.

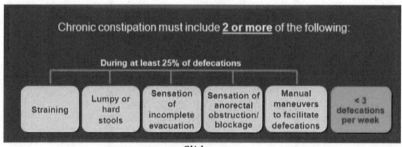

Slide 4

Now fiber, especially insoluble fiber - the kind you have in wheat bran - has long been heralded for its ability to bulk the stool, to make it bigger. But when you think about it logically, is making something bigger really the solution, when you're trying to pass it through a small hole? Packing the rectum with feces actually makes it harder to expel the fecal matter!

So using fiber to help constipation is analogous to adding more cars to fix a traffic jam! But that's not the only argument. People say: "Well, it also moistens the stool". Except... it doesn't!

It's been long known and well understood that stool moisture does not vary, regardless of how much fiber or how much water you consume. Fiber does not moisten the stool!

37

And while it's not technically a diagnostic feature of a constipation, bloating is a known issue that many people understand is related to excess consumption of fiber.

The reason for this is because it doesn't get digested in the small bowel, remember, that's the definition of fiber. It's not able to be digested. So it passes down to the large bowel, which has a large bacterial population.

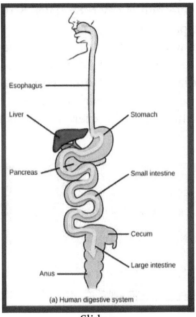

(a) Human digestive system

Slide 5

Then, these bacteria can ferment the fiber, especially the soluble fiber. They produce something called short chain fatty-acids, which is heralded as being one of the things which it provides health benefits through. But in the process of this, they also produce gases, such as hydrogen.

Given that the volume of the whole gastrointestinal tract is only about one liter, it only takes a relatively modest amount of gas production before you start feeling bloated and start having an element of abdominal pain.

And anybody who lived through the 1980s... anybody remember the bran craze? You can probably attest to that.

So what we're left with is that... when we look at their best evidence available:

- Fiber worsens constipation
- It causes bloating and
- It does absolutely nothing to moisten our feces.

So, how does this relate to low carbohydrate diets? Well, there's a lot of low carb foods that are actually high in fiber. So even though 45% of the fiber in the average Australian diet comes from breads and cereals, a lot of the food we replace it with, when we go on a low carbohydrate diet, are also high in fiber.

And: Some of the staples that we love! Like berries, cauliflower and almonds. They're in that high fiber group.

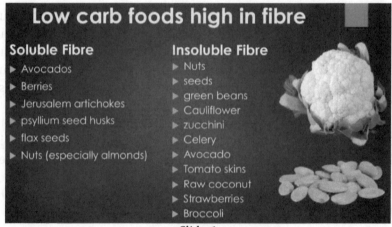

Slide 6

And if you understand that when they get metabolized in the colon, by the bacteria, they can produce gas and bloating - you can understand why, if you have a whole bag of nuts, you might feel a degree of discomfort down there.

So, some of you are probably looking at that, going: "You know what? I did have a big plate of cauliflower mash the other night and I did feel a bit funny overnight."

Let's turn our attention to something called the short chain fatty acids. Remember, once the fiber is fermented by bacteria, it produces these fatty acids. They're thought to offer some health benefits.

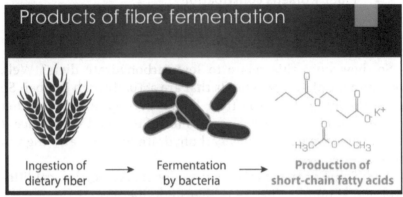

Slide 7

These bacteria allow the body to salvage energy from an otherwise unusable source, provided in the form of fats. Estimates vary widely, but it's commonly considered that about 5% of the energy we get from our diet, when we're eating an average diet, actually comes from these short chain fatty acids. Which are produced from fiber.

And it said that these short chain fatty acids nourish the cells that line our colon. They're called colonocytes. And this is thought to help improve conditions, like inflammatory bowel disease (IBD).

While it's true... this is a representation of some of the cells that line the colon:

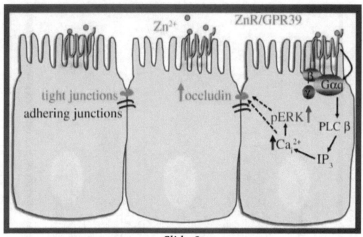

Slide 8

While these cells can use short chain fatty acids for energy, they only do so after converting them to ketones first! So, if ketones are produced from short chain fatty-acids, and that's beneficial - then isn't it logical that ketones in the circulation from being in nutritional ketosis, or in a ketogenic diet, would also be beneficial to these cells? They can still get to them.

In fact, the ketones in the circulation are probably even more effective because they're delivered to every colonocyte, not just those in which they're in direct contact with. This has actually being demonstrated in studies comparing enemas, giving short chain fatty acids, and giving ketones into the circulation.

And it's been shown that the ketones given in the circulation are more effective at treating the inflammation of IBD. Which might mean the short chain fatty-acids aren't so magical after all.

Even if they were, fiber isn't the only source of short chain fatty acids from gut bacteria. This graph here shows short chain fatty acid production between a plant-based diet, with lots of fiber - and an animal-based diet, with lots of amino a-cids.

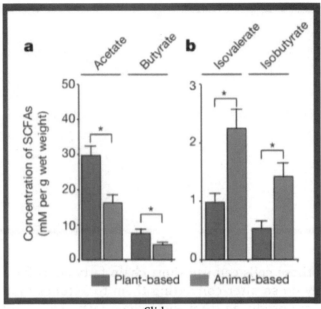
Slide 9

Here in red, (bars on the right sides) you can see that the short chain fatty acid production is actually higher on the animal-based diet than it is on the plant-based diet! So it would seem there's nothing uniquely beneficial about the production of short chain fatty acids from fiber at all.

Let's turn our attention to one of the other putative benefits of fiber in the diet. For example: That you can control your blood sugar levels. And when you take that in isolation, that's actually correct.

This graph here compares blood sugar levels between a diet recommended by the American Diabetes Association... yes, with all that spikes in blood sugar:

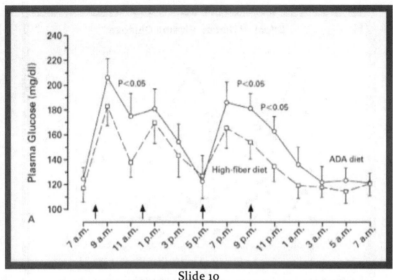

Slide 10

The Diabetic Association recommended diet. And below that line, a diet that's higher in fiber. So you can actually see that the high fiber diet actually does moderate the spikes in insulin, to a degree.

But the point that should probably be made is that: If you didn't eat all the carbohydrates in the first place, then you wouldn't need to worry about controlling the sugars with fiber!

Even with the fiber, if we convert it to our units, the blood sugar level still goes over 10. Additionally, if a diet that I was recommending for diabetes had blood sugar control like that, I'd probably start looking for another job!

So, let's have a look at this graph. This study was also published in the American Diabetes Association Journal. On the top, you can see a controlled diet with significant spikes in blood sugar level. On the bottom, you can see a diet that height looks massively better:

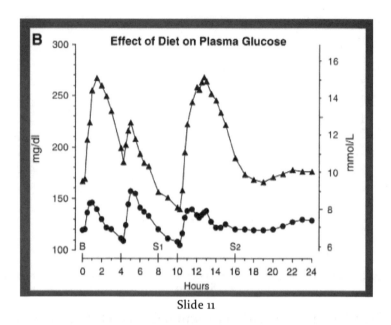

Slide 11

You know, far better than the diet that you just saw with
extra fiber added to it. Now, the diet on the bottom is what's
called a Low BAG Diet, this stands for *low biologically available
glucose diet.* I guess, you can't use the term low carb in a diabetes journal, huh?

Now, for a final thought on whether fiber is a necessary part
of a healthy diet, let's just look at a herbivore gut which has a
really large cecum, which is where fermentation of fiber occurs
- and compare it to a human gut:

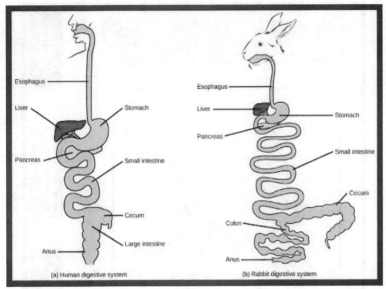

Slide 12

Clearly, you can see that our gastrointestinal tract just isn't set up to metabolize or process fiber in the way that herbivores are.

I'd like to now move on to the next section of my presentation, and have a look at something else that can cause gastric problems on a low-carb diet, And that's something called FODMAPs.

FODMAPs are carbohydrates, they are a group of short-chain carbohydrates with some common features. Firstly, they're poorly absorbed in the intestine. Because of that they get down to the colon where they can be fermented by the bacteria, again causing gas.

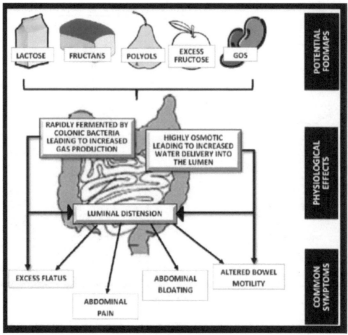

Slide 13

Much in the same way that happens with soluble fiber. Also, these FODMAPs, these particular carbohydrates, attract fluid due to a high level of osmotic activity, and that can lead to watery stools. Both of these symptoms are seen in a condition that we call irritable bowel syndrome (IBS).

As well as causing loose stools, FODMAPs can also cause constipation, something else which is seen in IBS. The way it does that is: When the bacteria have metabolized them, they produce methane. And methane gas has actually been shown to cause constipation.

And when people with IBS - repeated in lots of different studies - when they're put on a diet that's low in these FODMAPs, about 75% of them have significant improvements! I'd like to illustrate that point with a very interesting study published earlier this year.

There's a condition called non-celiac gluten sensitivity. These patients get gut symptoms when they eat foods that contain gluten. But when we test them for celiac disease, it all looks normal.

Now, the thing to understand is that foods that contain gluten also often contain something called fructans - and this is one of the FODMAPs. So, this study recruited patients with this non-gluten celiac sensitivity and gave them specially made bars.

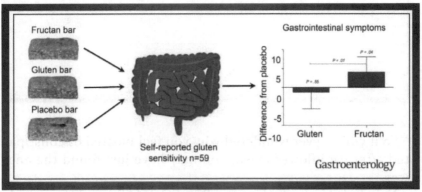

Slide 14

Some of them had fructan in them, some had gluten and some had neither. and what you can see on the right, is that their symptoms were far worse when they were given the fructans than when they were getting gluten. So it appears the diagnosis of non-celiac gluten sensitivity is in fact a problem with FODMAPs.

How does this relate to the low-carb diet? Because we don't tend to eat much wheat, right? True. But FODMAPs are found in a number of other foods, some of which are seen on a low carbohydrate diet. Unfortunately, this includes cauliflower - again, one of the staples which we also saw was high in fiber.

Fruits and Fruit Products	Vegetables and Vegetable Products	Milk Products	Grain and Starch-Based Foods	Legumes, Nuts, and Seeds	Others
Apple	Artichoke—globe	Cow's milk	Barley-, kamut-,	Cashews	Agave
Apricots	Artichoke—Jerusalem	Custard	rye-, and wheat-	Chickpeas	Fructose
Asian pears	Artichokes	Dairy desserts	based bread	Legumes (ie, red	Fructooligosaccharides
Blackberries	Asparagus	Evaporated milk	Cereal couscous	kidney beans,	Fruit juice concentrates
Boysenberry	Cauliflower	Goat's milk	Crackers	soy beans,	High-fructose corn
Cherries	Garlic	Ice cream	Croissants	borlotti beans)	syrup
Clingstone peach	Leek	Milk powder	Crumpets	Lentils	Honey
Custard apples	Mushroom	Sheep's milk	Gnocchi	Pistachios	Inulin
Mango	Onion	Sweetened	Muffins		Isomalt[a]
Nashi fruit	Shallot	condensed milk	Noodles		Maltitol[b]
Nectarines	Snow peas		Pasta		Polydextrose[d]
Peaches	Spring onion (white				Sorbitol[e]
Pears	part only)				
Plums	Sugar snap peas				
Prunes					
Persimmon					
Tamarillo					
Watermelon					
White peaches					

Slide 15

So if you've ever wondered why you feel bloated or constipated after cauliflower mash, you may have just found the answer.

Now let's have a look at the P in FODMAPs, and this stands for polyols, which represents artificial sweeteners called *sugar alcohols*. Because they essentially provide calorie free sweetness, polyols are used widely in a lot of low carb bars and sweets.

The problem is they're poorly absorbed, they attract water, they produce gas, they give you loose stools. And many people on low carb diets have suffered diarrhea as a consequence of having one too many Atkins bar.

Now I'd like to touch on what we call the microbiome. This reflects the colonies of bacteria or microbes that exist within the human body. But in particular, we're going to focus on those in the colon, in the large bowel.

It's often been said that we've got 10 times more bacteria than we do human cells. That's an exaggeration: When we actually look at the science, they do outnumber us by about 1.3. to one... but not quite 10 times.

So we're going to focus on the microbes right down at the bottom of this arrow here:

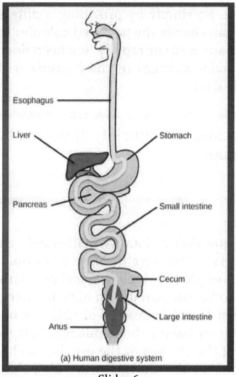

Esophagus

Liver

Stomach

Pancreas

Small intestine

Cecum

Large intestine

Anus

(a) Human digestive system

Slide 16

The question I want to specifically address is: Can these bacteria make us fat? Because that's what we've been hearing a lot about recently. Now, we've got more than a thousand different types of bacteria within our gut, but 90% of these come from one of two main groups:

The firmicutes phyla or the bacteroidetes. And the firmicutes phyla has actually been associated - in a number of studies - with obesity, while the bacteroidetes has been associated with weight loss.

Studies have demonstrates how, when you lose weight, the bacteroidetes actually increases. But the thing to understand about bacteria is, that they have very specific conditions for their growth.

Some prefer oxygen, some don't. Some like fiber, some don't... and so on. And the bacteria, if they like the conditions you give them, if they like the nutrition you provide them, they

49

will proliferate. So simply by providing a different source of nutrition, we can change the bacterial colonies in our gut.

And these changes occur rapidly. It's been documented that you can get major changes in the bacteria within your gut within a single day!

Diet rapidly and reproducibly alters the human gut microbiome

Lawrence A. David[1,2]†, Corinne F. Maurice[1], Rachel N. Carmody[1], David B. Gootenberg[1], Julie E. Button[1], Benjamin E. Wolfe[1], Alisha V. Ling[3], A. Sloan Devlin[4], Yug Varma[4], Michael A. Fischbach[4], Sudha B. Biddinger[3], Rachel J. Dutton[1] & Peter J. Turnbaugh[1]

Slide 17

But the big question is: Can we deliberately change the balance of bacteria to lose weight? Now, a key point here is that the bacteroidetes phyla (which is associated with weight loss) also happens to be associated with high-fat ketogenic diets.

This has been found in studies of children on this kind of diet, when they are having their epilepsy managed. So it becomes the case of the chicken or the egg: Is it a change in bacterial population? Or the change in the diet, that leads to the weight loss?

Back in 2006, there was this famous paper that was published that showed, that an obese microbiota could make mice fat. So they had some germ-free mice and they gave these germ-free mice some bacteria from some fat mice, and from some skinny mice.

And they actually found that the bacteria from the fat mice made these germ-free mice fatter. This is why: This graph here demonstrates short chain fatty acid production, comparing the two groups:

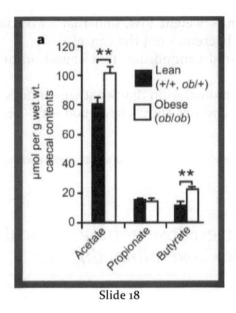

Slide 18

What you can see is that the obese bacteria led to an increased energy harvest, by way of producing more short chain fatty acids. But that doesn't mean that you can simply transplant bacteria in your colons to lose weight.

Firstly, the bacteria were transplanted into germ-free mice. There was no competition from other bacteria. It's highly unlikely that if you transplanted bacteria into a gut that had an existing colony, that it would do as well.

Secondly, the extra energy was derived from fiber. So if you're on a low fiber diet, then there would have been no finding. And the fact that their short chain fatty-acids are then converted into ketones - which, as we know, is an appetite suppressant...

That means that in the real world, when we're not on calorie controlled diets, when we're not just in a cage with a limited amount of food, that our volitional food intake becomes important. Thus, the ketones that are produced from the short chain fatty-acids probably would have had an appetite suppressant effect, and those mice would be predicted to then eat less.

So it's not clearly apparent that we can simply change our gut bacteria to lose weight. Far more likely is that changing our diet permits weight loss, and that's associated with the changing gut bacteria - not the cause!

It's the age-old conundrum. Is it causation or is it correlation?

As a final demonstration that what we eat does influence our gut bacteria - and not always in a good way - let's have a look at this study:

ARTICLE

doi:10.1038/nature25178

Dietary trehalose enhances virulence of epidemic *Clostridium difficile*

J. Collins[1], C. Robinson[2], H. Danhof[1], C. W. Knetsch[3], H. C. van Leeuwen[3], T. D. Lawley[4], J. M. Auchtung[1] & R. A. Britton[1]

Slide 19

Trehalose is a sugar composed of two glucose molecules. But it's fairly recent that it's been in our food supply, it was only approved for use in Australia in 2003, and that was after some Japanese scientists discovered a way to mass-produce it back in about 2000.

It's not very sweet, but it is very effective at lowering the freezing point of food. And because of that, it's used in a lot of things like ice cream. Now, the problem is that a particularly harmful bacteria called clostridium difficile is very fond of trehalose.

And the increased consumption since the early 2000s has been associated with an increase in a dangerous condition called pseudomembranous colitis associated with this bug. So what we eat changes our gut bacteria!

To conclude, I'd like to leave you with three key messages:
- Fiber is not a necessity for a healthy diet
- Secondly, even on a low carbohydrate diet, certain foods contain high levels of fiber or FODMAPs that can cause stomach upset, and you need to be aware of this. And finally:

- The whole concept of altering our microbiome for weight loss is a bridge too far with the current understanding of science.

Thank you.

Chapter 3
How lectins impact your health - From obesity to autoimmune disease

Good morning, my name is Dr. Paul Mason and I'm from Sydney. And today I'm going to talk to you about a protein that's found in plants, called lectins - and how they can have a massive impact on our health.

Understanding lectins, I believe, fills in a massive chasm in conventional medicine when it comes to treating a myriad of chronic diseases... and certainly for me, understanding their impact, has improved the care that I deliver to my patients.

As with all of my lectures, nothing contained here within should constitute personal medical advice.

So the story begins in 1976 in England when 9 school boys ate some kidney beans that had been soaked but not boiled.

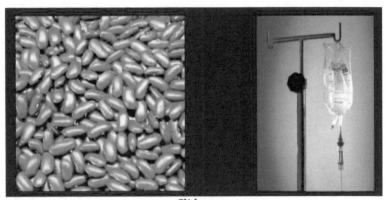

Slide 1

Within one and a half hours, all 9 of them ended up with profuse diarrhea and vomiting. Some of them had only consumed 4 kidney beans. And further illustrating the toxic potential of kidney beans is: A diet containing only 1% kidney beans will kill a rat in two weeks!

So the problem with uncooked kidney beans was considered so serious in England, back in this period, that the government started issuing written warning labels on uncooked kidney beans.

So then, that leaves us with the question: "What on earth is in uncooked kidney beans that will do that?" This is a kidney plant being here:

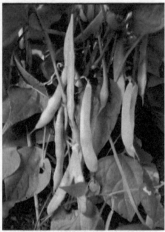
Slide 2

It doesn't have any claws, it can't run away. So it's pretty defenseless. Well, you'd be wrong! It's not at the complete mercy of any caterpillar that wants to come along, because it engages in some very potent chemical warfare. And the chemical warfare that plants use, one of them is called lectins.

The particular lectin contained in kidney beans is called phytohemagglutinin. In fact, there's over a hundred known sources of plant lectins and many of these are toxic to humans.

Each lectin is a protein with a unique structure, and it's a protein that has the ability to bind to carbohydrates. All of our cells in the body have these glycoproteins which protrude up from the cell membrane:

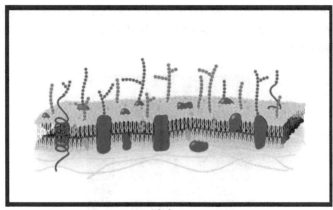

Slide 3

They contain a carbohydrate moiety on the end of it - and lectins can bind to that carbohydrate moiety. That means lectins can therefore bind to our human cells!

Now, lectins are resistant to cooking. In the case of red kidney beans, it's recommended that you should soak them for five hours and then boil them for at least 10 minutes to reduce the lectins to a less dangerous level.

As well as being heat stable, lectins are often very, very resistant to the normal digestive enzymes that we have lining our gut. And it's to the point where a lot of lectins provide no nutritional value at all, they're often excreteed completely unchanged.

And often, on the way through the intestinal tract, these unchanged lectins can often bind to the walls of our intestine and do significant damage, including killing the cells. So the way to think about it is: Our intestinal tract is a hollow tube from mouth to anus:

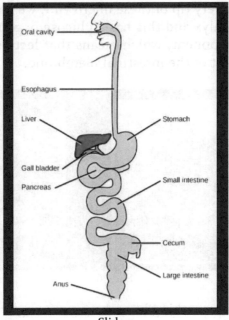

Slide 4

And ideally, it should allow absorption of nutrients across the wall, while not allowing entry of any toxins. And the lining of the intestinal tract has this basic structure. Firstly, there's a mucus layer on top (indicated in green here) and then beneath that, you've got these epithelial cells which are joined together, side by side, by what are called tight junctions.

And on top of the epithelial cells, you'll see that little fill layer. That's called micro villi.

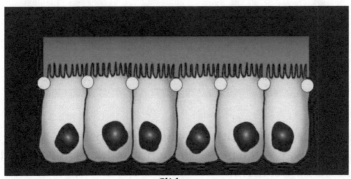

Slide 5

Now, on the very tip of these micro villi, we have something called a glycocalyx and this has a glucose or a sugar or a carbohydrate component, which means that lectins can actually bind to this part of the intestinal membrane.

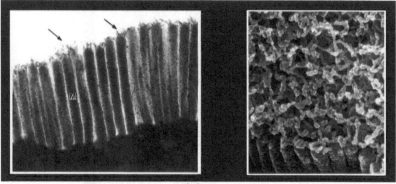
Slide 6

So if we take something like wheat germ agglutinin, that will actually bind to the internal lining of our gut and damage it. That causes something called leaky gut.

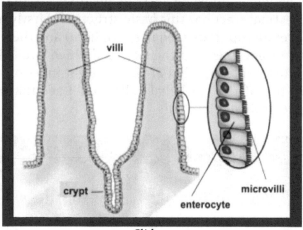
Slide 7

Now, once you've got this single layer of cells, if you then fold it in a way you can get these finger-like projections here, which we now call villi.

Now, coming back to the general function of the gastrointestinal tract: If we had a toxin like a lectin, hopefully it would pass straight through us without being absorbed. But occasionally, we can ingest a toxin and we have leaky gut or intestinal permeability, which allows the toxin to actually enter the body.

This is a graph that demonstrates the potential of these toxins, these lectins, to enter our body. Seven participants consumed 200 grams of peanuts. This test was actually measuring the amount of peanut lectin within their blood.

And you can see that within half an hour, the level started to rise - and within an hour, there was a significant amount of this lectin seen in the circulation.

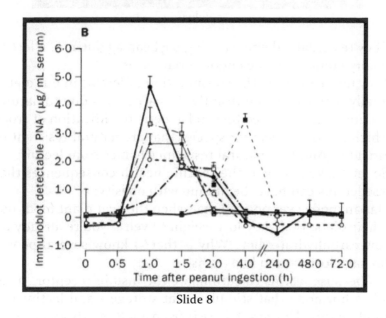

Slide 8

The ability of these lectins to bind to the surface of cells means that after entering our circulation, they can actually bind to cells in many different organs, depending on what particular affinity the leptin has for a particular kind of cell.

This image was done from a study, that was done on females with unexplained infertility. This is a sample of the endometrium, the lining of the uterus. And what you can actually see is indicated by the arrows:

59

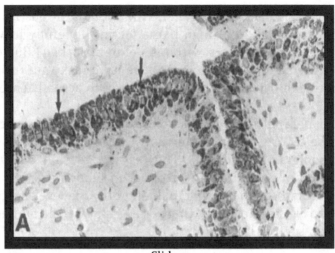

Slide 9

They're actually demonstrating soybean agglutinin, a lectin, actually bound to some endometrial tissue!

Now unfortunately, the consumption of lectins in our diet is actually increasing significantly. In part this is due to natural selection, selective breeding and genetic modification of crops - which tends to select for species that are natural resistant to pesticides. And that natural resistance comes from lectins.

So let's take a look at the specific health consequences that these lectins can have, beginning with obesity:

Has anybody ever noticed that when they cut plant foods out of their diets, that they lost weight? Even if you're already on a low carbohydrate diet? Why is that? I know several people who have lost over 10 kilograms!

It's because lectins can stimulate the insulin receptor. Insulin is a hormone that stimulates fat storage - and lectins can stimulate this! This graph here is from a 1983 study and it compared active fat storage between wheat germ agglutinin and insulin:

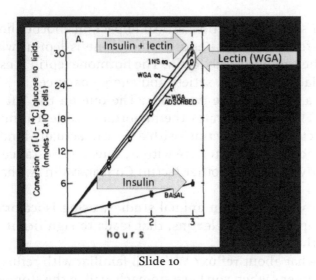

Slide 10

So down the bottom here, this is what happened to fat storage when insulin alone was given.

This is what happened to fat storage when insulin plus, a lectin in the form of wheat germ agglutinin, was given. You see the results in the upper arrow.

And this is what happened when you just give lectin alone: Middle arrow.

The point is that it stimulates the insulin receptor in a far more prolonged fashion than even does insulin. So this is a concern if you're trying to lose weight.

But it's not only wheat germ agglutinin that has this ability. In the same study, they actually looked at two other lectins as well. And you can see: "Ability to produce persistent lipogenesis." Creating fat.

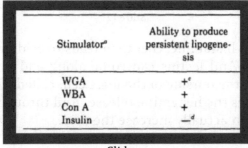

Stimulator[a]	Ability to produce persistent lipogenesis
WGA	+[c]
WBA	+
Con A	+
Insulin	−[d]

Slide 11

And it seems like lectin can also impact on another hormone critical to fat storage - and this hormone is leptin, with a P! Not to be confused with lectin. The hormone leptin is essential in regulating appetite, satiety and energy balance.

Have a look at these two mice: The one on the left has no leptin. That demonstrates the importance of leptin functioning effectively. And lectins -with a C - can actually bind to the leptin receptor and interfere with it, causing resistance. There is a study showing another lectin, Concanavalin A, that leads to leptin resistance.

When we test this in animal studies, using isocaloric diets that simply eliminate lectins, that leads to significant weight loss in the animals!

Now what about reflux? We're all familiar with reflux, that's what happens when you have stomach acid in the stomach that ascends up the esophagus. It's often called heartburn.

Well, you might be surprised to learn that lectins can also cause this because they can stimulate excess acid production. So this is a mast cell here and it can secrete a chemical called histamine.

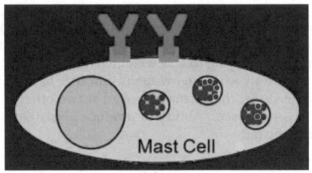

Slide 12

If it secretes histamine, that then leads to acid production in the stomach. And lectins can come along and bind to these molecules on the outside of the mast cell, called IG molecules, that stimulates the histamine release. And through this mechanism, you can actually increase the acid.

This is one study where it showed a dramatic reduction in the acid levels in the esophagus within six days of starting a low carbohydrate diet:

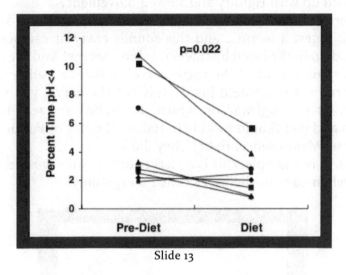

Slide 13

That's simply because when you go on a low carb diet, you often clear out the lectin-rich grains and cereals. So they actually had probes, down into the esophagus, that were sitting there for 24 hours and measuring the acid level constantly.

You can see that in a matter of six days, there was a significant reduction in the acidity within the esophagus. This is why symptoms of reflux often improve incredibly rapidly when we go on a plant-free diet.

Now, I'd like to make a very important point here: So far I've only talked about plant lectins but lectins. But lectins actually do exist in animal foods, and other foods, as well. The reason I'm only talking about plant lectins is that they're far more likely to be problematic.

That doesn't mean that animal-based lectins can't be problematic, it's just that they're so much less likely to do it.

There is a study looking at histamine release from 16 different lectins. The 4 that had the most significant response were all plant-based lectins! That's why I'm tending to focus on them.

Now, we'll turn our attention to a condition called Parkinson's disease. This is a movement disorder. I'm sure you've all heard of it, you're familiar with it: You end up with a tremor, you end up with rigidity and slowed movement.

There's evidence now that this is caused by lectins! You see, if you ingest a lectin... and this sounds crazy, it can actually ascend up to the brain by traveling along nerves! And the nerve in particular is called the vagus nerve. So theoretically - if that was true - if you would just simply cut the nerve, you would interrupt the highway on which the lectins are sent to the brain and you should be able to reduce the risk of Parkinson's disease. Makes sense, right? They did it!

This is an example, this is a picture of the two vagus nerves... and when you cut them, it's called a vagotomy.

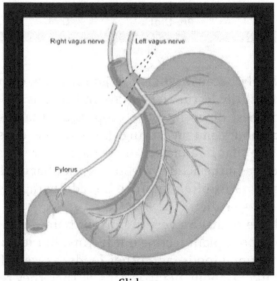

Slide 14

In one study published in 2015, they compared every patient in Denmark who had this procedure, between 1977 and 1995. This is what they found:

They found that by cutting the vagus nerves, the risk of developing Parkinson's disease dropped by 47%!

This is a more recent study that was able to actually confirm the mechanism: It was able to demonstrate that lectins were actually able to travel to the neurons in the brain (which are affected in Parkinson's disease).

This graphic here shows the ingested P lectin, sitting on top of a neuron in the brain that makes dopamine:

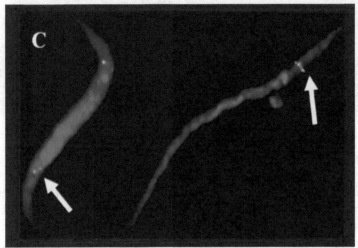

Slide 15

This is the problem in Parkinson's disease.

Now, I want to turn our attention to autoimmune disease: In autoimmune disease, the body attacks its own tissues. And the particular tissues attacked determine what specific autoimmune disease it is.

Because you've got a choice: There's heaps of them, more than you can poke a stick at.

Different examples of them might include different types of inflammatory arthritis. You might have pernicious anemia. You might even have multiple sklerosis, type 1 diabetes, inflammatory bowel disease, lupus and the list goes on.

But the point is that all autoimmune diseases are characterized by the body's immune system attacking itself. And one of the defining features is called *auto-antibodies*. So this y-shape structure here in the middle is what we call an antibody and it's one of the main features of the immune system:

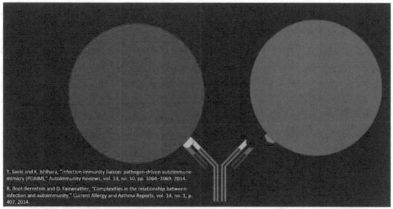

Y. Saeki and K. Ishihara, "Infection-immunity liaison: pathogen-driven autoimmune-mimicry (PDAIM)," Autoimmunity Reviews, vol. 13, no. 10, pp. 1064–1069, 2014.

R. Root-Bernstein and D. Fairweather, "Complexities in the relationship between infection and autoimmunity," Current Allergy and Asthma Reports, vol. 14, no. 1, p. 407, 2014.

Slide 16

Normally, antibodies are used to defend against foreign invaders. Pathogens. If you have a bacteria, the antibody will have a strong affinity for the bacteria - and when it attaches to it, that then stimulates or initiates an immune response that will lead to the eventual destruction of that bacteria.

If this was a healthy cell here: Well hopefully, that has no affinity for it. On the surface of the cell here, you see what's called an antigen. That's a particular molecular identifying feature, either on a cell or a bacteria. And the specificity of that antigen and the receptor on the antibody will depend whether they bind together or not.

In the case of autoimmune diseases, antibodies have receptors that can actually bind to healthy cells. And then, that can lead to your healthy tissues starting to be destroyed.

The presence of these auto-antibodies is actually what I use to diagnose autoimmune diseases. It's one of the major things I use, and there's over a 100 different antibodies that I can now test for - back home in Australia - when I'm trying to diagnose an autoimmune disease.

Now, leaky gut. This is intestinal permeability that allows lectins to enter into the circulation. Leaky gut is a key contributor to autoimmune disease and gluten is one of the major causes of leaky gut.

About 80% of the total protein contained within wheat is gluten. That's significant... but just from that one fact: It means that 80% of the protein is wheat is useless, so you're not getting as much protein as you think you are.

But the gluten is also very damaging to the intestinal barrier. This graph here demonstrates the intestinal barrier as assessed by something called trans epithelial electrical resistance (TEER):

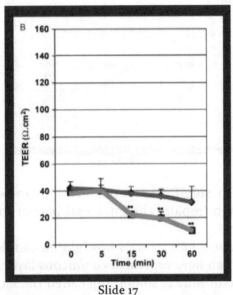

Slide 17

The higher the line, the better. The top line shows barrier function in celiac intestinal cells that haven't been exposed to gluten. When we expose them to gluten, this happens: It goes way down. You can see it happens rapidly, within 15 minutes. And in people with celiac disease, this increase in intestinal permeability will persist for up to a week!

But here's the thing that a lot of people don't know: It's not only celiacs who are affected by gluten!

This top line here is non-celiacs cells, not exposed to gluten - this one here non-celiacs cells exposed to gluten:

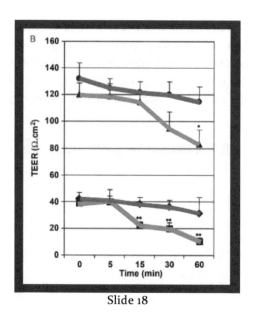

Slide 18

There's still a significant impediment to intestinal barrier function. Gluten impairs the intestinal barrier in everybody - not just celiacs!

Now, let's have a look exactly how gluten can do this. So the top layer in green here represents a mucous layer, and the bottom layer here in blue is something called the lamina propria. This is the tissue layer of the intestines where the immune system lives. You've got blood vessels and lymphatic vessels and a few other things kicking around there.

And this here is gluten on the upper left:

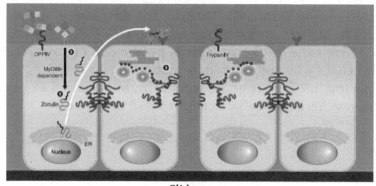

Slide 19

Now, when it gets ingested, it can get broken down partially into these smaller parts called gliadin. But no further. And this gliadin then can bind to a special receptor called CXC-R3.

Once it binds to that, that leads to signaling within the cell... leads to the production of a molecule called zonulin. This zonulin can then come and act on a receptor which leads to the breakdown of these proteins here, called the tight junction (or gap junction), which actually hold the cells together. And when that gets disrupted, the cells are able to physically separate - this is what causes leaky gut! This is what leaky gut is!

And then, these lectins that have been ingested - as well as any bacteria that might exist in the intestines - can actually pass between the cells and get down to the lamina propria, where it gets exposed to the immune

Now, because lectins are essentially foreign particles, we often mount an immune response to get them. So we often end up developing antibodies that will target them.

Let's say here in purple (left), that that's a lectin - and if you have a look at the antigen on the surface in green (small unit below), you can see that it's the same, as part of an antigen on a healthy cell:

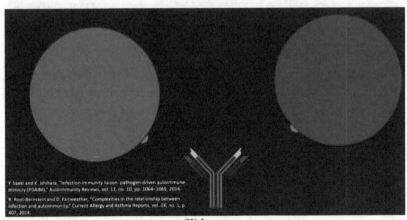

Y. Saeki and K. Ishihara, "Infection-immunity liaison: pathogen-driven autoimmune mimicry (PDAIM)," Autoimmunity Reviews, vol. 13, no. 10, pp. 1064-1069, 2014.

R. Root-Bernstein and D. Fairweather, "Complexities in the relationship between infection and autoimmunity," Current Allergy and Asthma Reports, vol. 14, no. 1, p. 407, 2014.

Slide 20

That means: If we develop an antibody response against a lectin, we can also develop an antibody response against a healthy cell. And this is called molecular mimicry - and this is thought to underpin most autoimmune disease!

(...)

Now, one of the conditions that's linked to type 1 diabetes is gluten consumption. So if you consume gluten, it's been shown that your risk of developing type 1 diabetes, Hashimoto's, thyroiditis, these other clusters of autoimmune diseases, is significantly increased.

This recent study encapsulates that risk with "maternal gluten consumption", looking at the risk of developing type 1 diabetes in offspring:

Maternal gluten intake, by percentile*	Hazard ratio (95% CI) of type 1 diabetes diagnosis in offspring
Continuous intake, per 10 g/day increse	1.31 (1.001 to 1.72)
10%	1.00 (reference)
10-20%	1.06 (0.57 to 1.99)
20-50%	1.31 (0.75 to 2.30)
50-80%	1.46 (0.82 to 2.60)
80-90%	1.81 (0.93 to 3.53)
≥90%	2.00 (1.02 to 4.00)
P_{trend}	0.016

Slide 21

They looked at over a 100,000 pregnancies in Denmark and what they found was there was a reliable linear increased risk of type 1 diabetes with gluten consumption. And for the highest group of gluten consumption, the risk of your offspring developing type 1 diabetes was doubled!

And then we have papers like this, which indicate that commencing a gluten-free diet soon after diagnosis of type 1 diabetes can significantly alter the prognosis. This study looked at what happened to a boy who was placed on a strict gluten-free diet soon after diagnosis of type 1 diabetes, and it compared him to a group of 21 other children as a control:

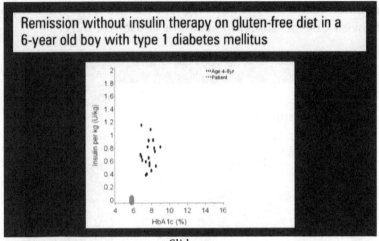

What you can see: Here he is down in red, his insulin level, his insulin usage, was far far less - and his blood sugar control was far far better. It had him in the sub 6 group, rarefied air. And his diabetes was still in remission 20 months later, when this study was actually published.

Now, just a little bit of a semi related point I'd like to raise: We cannot assume that only children develop type 1 diabetes. We don't call it that in adults, we use the "term latent autoimmune diabetes of adulthood", which is a pretty cumbersome name - but it's essentially the same. It's diabetes of autoimmune origin!

In fact, up to 14 percent of cases of "type 2 diabetes", which are diagnosed in adults, actually have an autoimmune component. And this is huge! Because it means there's a potential intervention that we might be able to do for these other people that we're missing out on.

Unfortunately, we very, very rarely test for autoimmune diabetes in adults, despite the fact that the chances are more than 1 in 10 of type 2 diabetics actually having this condition. And it doesn't matter if you're overweight and have other metabolic risk factors, you still could have this autoimmune type of adult onset diabetes.

So it's probably time to pause for a moment and ask why not everybody has an autoimmune disease? Because we've all consumed lectins in the past, right? So I find it helpful to apply the Swiss Cheese model of accident causation here:

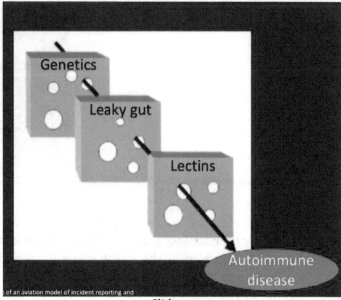

Slide 23

That states that accidents only happen when deficiencies in the defenses line up. So if we have a think about autoimmune diseases

- you need to pick the wrong parents
- you probably need to have some aspect of intestinal permeability, which may or may not be triggered by lectin consumption. And then
- you may also need to be consuming lectins or have some other kind of antigenic stimulus, like certain bacteria within your gut.

So unless all of those three line up, then chances are you probably won't develop an autoimmune disease. But for people that have picked the wrong parents, those next two layers become very important.

Let's pay a bit more attention to intestinal permeability or leaky gut now. This chart here was derived from a genome Association study looking at you inflammatory bowel disease:

72

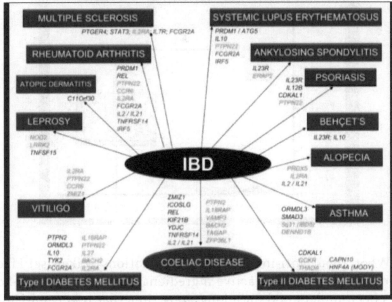

Slide 24

It found that having inflammatory bowel disease, or the genetics for it, increased the risk of 23 other conditions, most of them autoimmune diseases. So this should suggest that there's something about inflammatory bowel disease which is inherently associated with increased intestinal permeability that is problematic in autoimmune disease.

Let's start with a few factors of things that we can actually do to reduce, or increase, intestinal permeability, other risk factors.

Alcohol's a big one! So clearly here, you see that intestinal permeability is far higher consuming ethanol, than not:

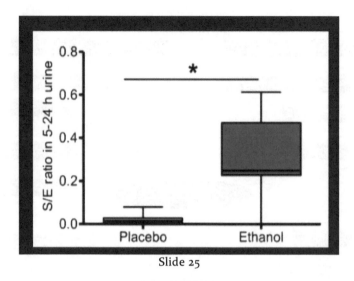

Slide 25

What about anti-inflammatory medications? Likewise! Like diclofenac, this is the active ingredient found in Voltaren. So it's been understood for a long, long time that taking anti-inflammatory medication increases intestinal permeability.

And to add insult to injury: These are the medications that doctors often prescribe to people with joint pain... in a group of arthritis, called the seronegative spondyloarthropathies, or even rheumatoid arthritis... these other conditions that as a rootcause will often have intestinal permeability contributing.

Now, let's have a look at our processed foods. They're full of a myriad of ingredients, they're always homogenized. And the reason is because they contain emulsifiers.

This study here - it was done in mice - but it actually compared a couple of emulsifiers at one percent of their food intake, so it wasn't big. Compared to the amount of emulsifiers that an average person on a processed food diet consumes, this is actually quite modest.

But what you can see, the addition of emulsifiers, in the second or the third column here, leads to a significant thinning of the mucus (shown in the green layer in the middle) and it actually allows increased bacterial penetration of the mucus:

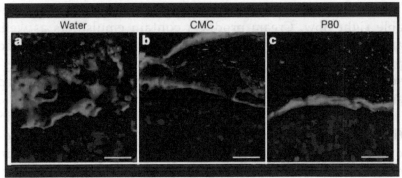

Slide 26

So you can see the red dots, they are the bacteria (on the right picture, theyre the small dots above the middle mucus layer). They're now able to get very close to the intestinal wall.

And if we actually have a look at what the consequences are of this... in the same study, we find that exposure to the emulsifiers increased volitional food intake. We didn't tell the mice to eat more - they just did! The second and third columns there:

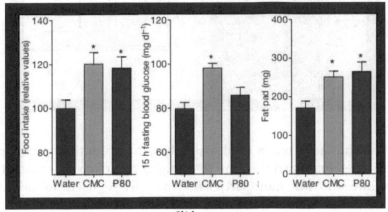

Slide 27

Predictably, this then led to a significant increase in fasting blood glucose levels. And, perhaps even more predictably, the mice got fatter. The authors of this paper basically said "It was emulsifier-induced metabolic syndrome." So anybody's still clinging to the *calories in calories out* hypothesis?

But even those on a ketogenic diet shouldn't get too comfortable right now. Cream products contain emulsifiers as well, and they're also found in things like coconut cream too - so please check your labels. They're not often stated, like polysorbate 80... it's nice if they say that, but it's often just listed as e433. So check your labels if you're having processed foods.

Polyethylene glycol is another substance that can really thin the mucus layer. That's often used as an anti-foaming food additive, or it's often used to manage or treat constipation in drugs called Movicol, that's actually made of polyethylene glycol.

In this study here, we can see what happened when you add polyethylene glycol to a sugar mixture in mice. See how it impacts a thickness of the mucus layer there (right bar):

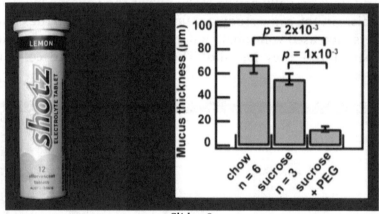

Slide 28

Another additive in food which has the potential to damage the intestinal barrier is one that might surprise you - that's titanium dioxide nanoparticles. Now, we're used to talking about titanium dioxide in sunscreens when we worry about it. But you can probably relax because it doesn't seem to penetrate to the deeper layers of the skin to the dermis, where it can actually interact with the immune system.

But if you eat it, that's a different story - and it's an approved food additive! And you might well be eating it, it's often in sweets and chewing gums. Studies have actually shown (in animals) that regular consumption for a period of 10 days will actually lead to detectable accumulations in organs.

What we've got here is a stick of sugar-free and gluten-free chewing gum.

INGREDIENTS: SORBITOL, GUM BASE, MALTITOL, MALTITOL SYRUP, XYLITOL, NATURAL FLAVORS, GUARANA (WITH NATURAL CAFFEINE), BACOPA MONNIERA, GINKGO BILOBA, GUM ARABIC, TITANIUM DIOXIDE, SUCRALOSE, RESINOUS GLAZE, CARNUBA WAX, SOY LECITHIN, VINPOCETINE, AND BHT (TO MAINTAIN FRESHNESS).

MANUFACTURED IN THE USA. © 2012 THINK GUM LLC.   222065-A

Slide 29

And, as an aside, it's so effective at penetrating the gut barrier, that drug companies use it for drug delivery... they try and complex a drug molecule with a nanoparticle, because they know the nanoparticle can actually get past the intestinal wall.

Now we move to pesticides. Pesticides of all sorts have been associated with a whole lot of autoimmune disorders, neurological defects, developmental disorders. And what we can see here is a study on pesticides. So you can see there in green (the fine lines), these are tight junctions of proteins that hold the epithelial cells together:

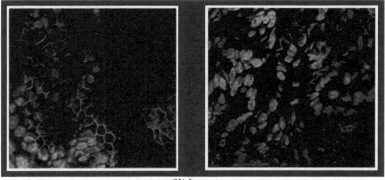

Slide 30

They're being highlighted by something called immunofluorescence. And this is a sample that hasn't been exposed to pesticides - and the picture on the right shows a sample from a mouse that has been exposed to pesticides. The tight junctions are gone!

And associated with this loss of tight junctions is increased passage of bacteria into the circulation.

So this is from the same study. This graph demonstrates the percentage of rats following pesticide exposure, who had different classes of bacteria in their circulation. The gray bars demonstrate the rats exposed to pesticides and the white bars demonstrate the rats who weren't:

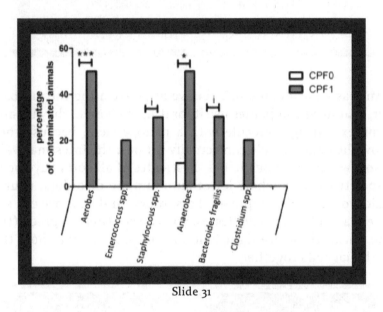

Slide 31

Here's the problem: Many of our foodstuffs are actually contaminated with pesticide residues.

This is one that might surprise a lot of people... we've all heard about people moving to the mountains and their inflammatory bowel disease got better, or something like that. And pollution may be there to blame.

Particularly, the really small particles called the PM10s. They've actually been shown to increase gut permeability. In this graph here, in control mice, we have mice exposed to PM10:

78

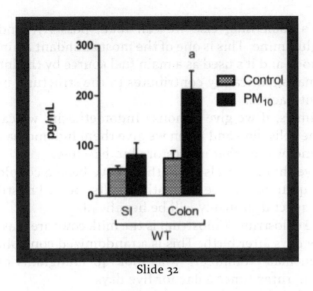

Slide 32

You can see, there's a significant increase in intestinal permeability, especially in the colon. The reason it's worse in the colon is probably because the residue spends the longest time in that part of the gastrointestinal tract. They can also induce free radical damage, which then has a whole another list of consequences in terms of oxidative stress and free radical production.

What about chemicals found in plastic? You've all probably heard of BPA, and we know that BPA is damaging to the gut lining. But it's being taken out of the the food packaging now, right? So that's got to be a good thing.

Well, it's being replaced by something called BPS. It basically has the same effect - we think. Except, it hasn't really been studied. But now, 80% of Americans actually have detectable levels of BPS in their urine. So maybe stay away from plastics.

Now, let's have a look at things that you can do, things that are good. The consumption of fats has actually been shown to significantly improve the function of the mucus layer in the intestines. And the effect was significant. So when we compared it, we had 200 nanometer spheres and we measured the passage of those across a barrier.

The consumption of fats immediately preceding that, reduced the passage by at least 10 times and possibly more than 100 times!

There's something else we can take, possibly. And that's called glutamine. This is one of the most abundant amino acids in the body and it's used as a main fuel source by the intestinal cells. That significantly contributes to the structural integrity of the interacites.

In animals, if we give a mouse Indomethacin, we can see a lot of the cells die - and when we give them Indomethacin plus glutamine, we see that it's restored to baseline.

So as yet human trials - and there have been a couple - they haven't quite had those dramatic results, but... I'm still waiting. I suspect it probably will be beneficial.

Bovine colostrum: Colostrum is the milk cows are making the first few days after birth. This is a randomized controlled trial on seven male volunteers who took 40 milligrams of Indomethacin, three times a day for five days.

What they found was that before they took Indomethacin, and after they took Indomethacin - if they had colostrum - there was no change in their intestinal permeability.

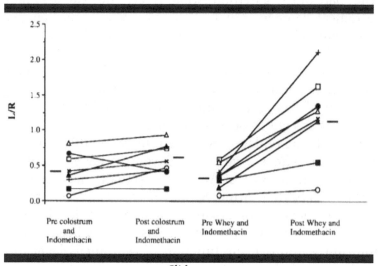

Slide 33

But if they didn't take the colostrum and they took a surrogate, a whey protein, then there was a significant increase. And it's thought to be that there's growth factors in the colostrum...

in particular, transforming growth factor beta, which is thought to support the intestinal wall.

Now, by definition, lectins can bind to sugars because they're carbohydrate-protein. So the theory is that, perhaps, if we're consuming lectins, we can consume sugars at the same time - and these sugars will serve as a decoy and bind to the lectins before they can hit our intestinal wall and do the damage.

What you can see in a study on mice, is that if they were given a lectin on its own, there's a significant increase in intestinal permeability. But when they gave a co-consumption of sugar plus the lectin, the damage was reduced.

There's also theories that giving glucosamine supplement will do the same So we can actually do a decoy.

Now, the really interesting thing to consider is that if you're a vegetarian on a low carbohydrate diet, then you may actually be getting more damage from the lectins.

Now, lecithin is a unique substance: This is often used as a natural emulsifier in foods - but it's a good guy. It actually contains something called phosphatidylcholine, and more than 70% of the phospholipids in our mucous membrane is made as phosphatidylcholine.

Orally ingested lecithin has actually been shown to adhere to the mucous layer and strengthen it. In one randomized control trial, that led to a more than 50 percent improvement in symptoms, in more than 90 % of patients with inflammatory bowel disease.

And this was in a population that was refractory to steroids and other medications. In fact, 80% of patients who were on steroids were able to have them withdrawn because of the lecithin.

Now, we've already seen a significant association between bacterial populations in the gut and intestinal permeability. So the question is: Well, can we replace... can we supplement with bacterial populations in the form of probiotics? And several strains of bacteria have actually been shown to be beneficial to the intestinal lining.

This includes lactobacillus plantarum which is found in a medical-grade probiotic supplement called VSL#3, that we often use in inflammatory bowel disease. One of the issues is, though, the need to nourish any introduced bacteria.

If the food supply or the nutrients available for the bacteria which we introduce is not favorable to it, it's likely to be outcompeted by other bacteria. That just means that we're going to need to have a continual delivery.

Now, as you know, there's some debate about whether we should have dairy foods. And a lot of the debate goes around whether we should have A1 or A2 proteins. So basically, A1 protein - which is found in some milks - can lead to the formation of a peptide called BCM7. And this has certain opiate-type effects.

It can bind to opiate receptors in the brain, possibly lead to cognitive dysfunction. And it's thought that it might also cause intestinal inflammation and several other things. There are some studies that actually show, comparing A1 and A2 milks... that eliminating the A1 protein led to a reduction in systemic inflammation and improving cognitive performance and several other things.

But there is a take-home point here: Because (putting that to one side) both the milks still led to a low-grade inflammatory response, the type of which is often seen in conditions what we call atopy - allergic type conditions, asthmatic type conditions.

So it's probably reasonable here to err on the side of caution: If you have a genetic susceptibility for developing allergies or autoimmune disease, then avoiding cow's milk for the first period of your life is certainly highly recommended, and possibly ongoing avoidance.

Just to wind up. The question is: With all of this theory, does avoiding these plant-based lectins actually help auto immune conditions? And the answer is: Yes!

There was a study that was published in 2017 and it looked at a cohort of 15 patients with inflammatory bowel disease. And remember: Inflammatory bowel disease was at the center of this diagram of all the other autoimmune diseases.

The average duration of inflammatory bowel disease in the study participants was 19 years! And 7 of the 15 actually relied on expensive treatments, what we call *biological therapy monoclonal antibodies*, to try to help control their disease.

They were placed on a diet that was called The Autoimmune Protocol: So they avoided gluten, refined sugar, grains, legumes, nightshade vegetables... because they carry a lot of lectins, a lot of people don't realize that. That means your potato, your bell peppers, your eggplants, tomatoes, chilies - very rich in lectins.

We cut out the nightshades. No dairy, no eggs, no coffee, no alcohol, no nuts, no seeds. No food additives. They also gave them a little bit of lifestyle advice, you know: Optimize your sleep, exercise a little bit.

So what were the results? Well, 11 of the 15 subjects had clinical remission by six weeks - and they maintained it for the duration of the study!

Week 0 versus 11 Results	n	Week 0	Week 11	P
FC (μg/g), mean (SD)	6	471 (562)	112 (104)	0.12
Baseline FC >50 μg/g, mean (SD)	4	701 (563)	139 (113)	0.09
CRP (mg/L), mean (SD)	9	3.9 (5.2)	3.4 (5.3)	0.82
Albumin (g/dL), mean (SD)	10	4.1 (0.4)	3.9 (0.4)	0.36

Slide 34

Remember: The average duration of inflammatory bowel disease entering this study was 19 years! Now, by virtue of the small study size, the laboratory measurements didn't reach statistical significance. But they did show a trend for improvements.

Take for example fecal calprotectin (FC), this is a marker of bowel inflammation they get shed off into the feces, and it's a very reliable test of inflammatory bowel disease. In actual fact, it's one of my preferred tests for this condition that I do in the clinic.

The average reduction was from 475 to 112! Now, it didn't reach statistical significance by virtue of the small sample size.

But certainly, reductions like that are what I'd consider clinically significant. And these kind of results mirror the results that I actually see in my patients.

Thank you!

Sources Chapter 1

Slide 1 of video presentation (Shown as slide 1 in this printversion):

Red Kidney Bean Poisoning in the UK: An Analysis of 50 Suspected Incidents between 1976 and 1989.
J.C. Rodhouse, C.A. Haugh, D. Roberts and R.J. Gilbert
Epidemiology and Infection, Vol. 105, No. 3 (Dec. 1990), pp. 485-491

The effect of the consumption of red kidney beans (Phaseolus vulgaris) on the growth of rats and the implications for fuman populations.
McPherson LL.
J R Soc Health. 1990 Dec; 110 (6): 222-6.

Do dietary lectins cause diseaseThe evidence is suggestive - and raises interesting possibilities for treatment.
D L J Freed.
BMJ. 1999 Apr 17; 318 (7190): 1023-1024.

Slide 2 (Shown as slide 2):

Castor bean toxicity reexamined: a new perspective.
Rauber A, Heard J.
Vet Hum Toxicol. 1985; 27: 498-502

Slide 3:

Lectins in the United States diet: a survey of lectins in commonly consumed foods and a review of the literature.
Nachbar M.S., Oppenheim J.D.
The American Journal of Clinical Nutrition. 1980. 33 (11), 2338-2345.

Dietary lectins as disease causing toxicants.
Hamid R., Masood A.
Pak J Nutr., 2009, 8, 293-303.

Slide 4:

Mislovičová D, Gemeiner P, Kozarova A & Kožár T (2009):
Relevance of exogenous plant lectins in biomedical diagnostics.
Biologia, 6 4 (1), 1-19.

Slide 7:

Pusztai A.
Plant Lectins; p.272
Cambridge University Press; Cambridge, UK: 1991.

Slide 8 (Shown as 4):
Anselmi, L. et al. (2018)
Ingestion of subtthreshold doses of environmental toxins induces ascending Parkinsonism in the rat.
NPJ Parkinson's Disease, 4 (1).

Slide 11 (Shown as 6):

Pellegrina, C. et al. (2009).
Effects of wheat germ agglutinin on human gastrointestinal epithelium: insights from an experimental model of immune/epithelial cell interaction.
Toxicology and Applied Pharmacology, 237 (2), 146-153.

Three-dimensional ultrastructure of the brush border glycocalyx in the mouse small intestine: a high resolution scanning electron microscopic study.
Horiuchi K, Naito I, Nakano K, Nakatani S, Nishida K, Taguchi T, Ohtsuka A.
Arch Histol Cytol. 2005; 68(1): 51-6.

The filamentous brush border glycocalyx, a mucin-like marker of enterocyte hyper-polarization.
Maury J, Nicoletti C, Guzzo-Chambraud L, Maroux S.
Eur J Biochem. 1995 Mar 1; 228 (2): 323-31

Slide 15 (Shown as 8):

Identification of intact peanut lectin in peripheral venous blood.
Wang Q, Yu LG, Campbell BJ, Milton JD & Rhodes JM.
The Lancet. 1998, 352 (9143), 1831-1832.

Slide 16 (Shown as 9):

Marziali M, Venza M, Lazzaro S, Lazzaro A, Micossi C, Stolfi VM.
Gluten-free diet: a new strategy for management of painful endometriosis related symptoms?
Miverva Chir. 2012; 67 (6): 499-504

Rogers, PA et al
Research Priorities for Endometriosis.
Reproductive Sciences. 2016, 24(2), 202-226.

Klentzeris LD, Bulmer JN, Li T-C, Morrison L, Warren A & Ian Douglas Cooke.
Lectin binding of endometrium in women with unexplained infertility.
Fertility and Sterility. 1991, 56 (4), 660-667.

de Oliveira JTA.
Changes in organs and tissues induced by feeding of purified kidney bean (Phaseolus vulgaris) lectins.
Nutrition Research, Volume 8, Issue 8. August 1988, pp. 943-947.

Do dietary lectins cause disease?
Freed DL.
BMJ 1999, 318: 1023-1024

Gabor F, Klausegger U, Wirth M.
The interaction between wheat germ agglutinin and other plant lectins with prostate cancer cells Du-145.
Int J Pharm. 2001, 221: 35-47

Geleff S, Bock P.
Pancreatic duct glands. II. Lectin binding affinities of ductular epithelium, ductular glands and Brunner glands.
Histochemistry. 1984, 80: 31-38.

Pusztai A, Clarke EMW, Grant G, King TP.
The toxicity of Phaseolus vulgaris lectins. Nitrogen balance and immuno-chemical studies.
J. Sci. Food Agric. 1981; 32: 1037-1046.

Slide 17:

Macedo M, Oliveira C & Oliveira C.
Insecticidal Activity of Plant Lectins and Potential Application in Crop Protection.
Molecules. 2015, 20 (2), 2014-2033.

Slide 18 (Shown as 10):

Shechter Y.
Bound lectins that mimic insulin produce persistent insulin-like activities.
Endocrinology. 1983 Dec; 113 (6); 1921-6.

Slide 20:

Kamikubo Y et al.
Contribution of leptin receptor N-linked glycans to leptin binding.
Biochem J. 2008; 410 (3): 595-604

Slide 23 (Shown as 12):

Pramond E et al.

Potato lectin activates basophils and mast cells of atoptic subjects by its interaction with core chitobiose of cell-bound non-specific immunoglobulin.
Clin Exp Immunol. 2007 Jun; 148 (3): 391-401.

Haas H et al.
Dietary lectins can induce in-vitro release of IL-4 and IL-13 from human basophils.
European Journal of Immunology. 1999, 29(3), 918-927.

Slide 24 (Shown as 13):

Austin GL, Thiny MT, Westman EC, Yancy WS & Shaheen NJ.
A very low carbohydrate diet improves gastroesophageal reflux and its symptoms.
Digestive Diseases and Sciences. 2006, 51 (8), 1307-1312.

Slide 25:

Pramond SN et al.
Potato lectin activates basophils and mast cells of atopic subjects by its interaction with core chitobiose of cell-bound non-specific immunoglobulin E.
Clin Exp Immunol. 2007 Jun; 148(3): 391-401.

Haas H et al.
Dietary lectins can induce in-vitro release of IL-4 and IL-13 from human basophils.
European Journal of Immunology. 1999, 29(3), 918-927.

Slide 26:

Anselmi L et al.
Ingestion of subthreshold doses of environmental toxins induces ascending Parkinsonism in the rat.
NPJ Parkinsons's Disease. 2018, 4 (1)

Slide 27 (Shown as 14):

Svensson E. et al.
Vagotomy and subsequent risk of Parkinson's disease.
Annals of Neurology. 2015, 78 (4), 522-529.

Slide 29 (Shown as 15):

Zheng J, et al.

Dietary plant lectins appear to be transported from the gut to gain access to and alter dopaminergic neurons of Caenorhabditis elegans, a potential etiology of Parkinson's Disease.
Frontiers in Nutrtion. 2016, 3.

Slide 31 (Shown as 16):

Saeki A & Ishihara K.
Infection-immunity liaison: pathogen-driven autoimmune-mimicry (PDAIM)
Autoimmunity Reviews. 2014, vol. 13, no. 10, pp. 1064-1069.

Root-Bernstein R & Fairweather D.
Complexities in the relationship between infection and autoimmunity.
Current Allergy and Asthma Reports. 2014, vol. 14, no. 1, p. 407.

Lis J, Jarzab A, Witkowska D.
Molecular mimicry in the etiology of autoimmune diseases.
Advances in Hygiene and Experimental Medicine (online). 2012, vol. 66, pp. 475-491.

Slide 32:

Haupt-Jorgenson M et al.
Possible Prevention of Diabetes with a gluten-free diet.
Nutrients. 2018, 10 (11), 1746.

Slide 33 (Shown as 17+18):

Drago S et al.
Gliadin, zonulin and gut permeability: Effects on celiac and non-celiac intestinal mucosa and intestinal cell lines.
Scandinavian Journal of Gastroenterology. 2006, 41 (4), 408-419.

Lammers KM et al.
Gliadin induces an increase in intestinal permeability and zonulin release by binding to the chemokine receptor CXCR3.
Gastroenterology. 2008, 135 (1), 194-204. E3.

Slide 34 (Shown as 19):

Sturgeon C & Fasano A.
Zonulin, a regulator of epithelial and endothelial barrier functions, and its involvement in chronic inflammatory diseases.
Tissue Barriers. 2016, 4:4, e1251384.

Slide 36:

Uhlig's Corrosion Handbook: Second Edition Revie, W. et al. 2000.
Microbial degradation of polymeric materials.

Cordain L et al.
Modulation of immune function by dietary lectins in rheumatoid arthritis.
British Journal of Nutrition. 2000, 83 (03), pp. 207-217.

Slide 37:

Tanaka S et al.
Lipopolysaccharide accelerates collagen-induced arthritis in association
with rapid and continuous production of inflammatory mediators and anti-
type II collagen antibody.
Microbiol Immunol. 2013 Jun; 57 (6): 445-54

Slide 38:

Wang X, Quinn PJ & Yan A.
Kdo2-lipid A: Structural diversity and impact on immunopharmacology.
Biological Reviews. 2014, 90 (2), 408-427.

Slide 39:

Wu GD et al.
Linking long-term dietary patterns with gut microbial enterotypes.
Science. 2011, 334 (6052), 105-108.

D'Hennezel et al.
Total lipopolysaccharide from the human gut microbiome silences toll-like
receptor signaling.
mSystems. 2017, 2 (6)

Slide 40:

Xie G et al.
Ketogenic diet poses a significant effect on imbalanced gut microbiota in
infants with refractory epilepsy.
World Journal of Gastroenterology. 2017, 23 (33), 6164-6171

Ley RE, Turnbaugh PJ, Klein S & Gordon JI.
Human gut microbes associated with obesity.
Nature, 2005.

Slide 41 (Shown as 21):

Antvorskov JC et al.
Association between maternal gluten intake and type 1 diabtes in offspring:
National prospective cohort study in Denmark.

BMJ. 2018, k3547

Slide 42 (Shown as 22):

Sildorf SM, Fredheim S, Svensson J & Buschard K.
Remission without insulin therapy on gluten-free diet in a 6-year old boy
with type 1 diabetes mellitus.
Case Reports. 2012, June 1, bcr0220125878-bcr0220125878

Slide 43:

Pozzilic P, Pieralice S.
Latent Autoimmune Diabetes in Adults: Current Status and New Horizons.
Endocrinol Metab (Seoul). 2018, Jun 33(2): 147-159

Slide 44 (Shown as 23):

Ferroli P et al.
Application of an aviation model of incident reporting and investigation to
the neurosurgical scenario: method and preliminary data.
Neurosurg Focus. 2012 Nov; 33(5): E7

Slide 45 (Shown as 24):

Lees CW et al.
New IBD genetics: common pathways with other diseases.
Gut. 2011, 60 (12), 1739-1753

Slide 46 (Shown as 25):

Elamin E et al.
Ethanol impairs intestinal barrier function in humans through mitogen ac-
tivated protein kinase signaling.
PloS One. 2014, 9 (9): e107421

Slide 47:

Wallace JL et al.
Proton pump inhibitors exacerbate NSAID-induced small intestinal injury
by inducing dysbiosis.
Gastroenterology. 2011, 141 (4), 1314-1322. e5.

Slide 48 (Shown as 26):

Chassaing B et al.
Dietary emulsifiers impact the mouse gut microbiota promoting colitis and
metabolic syndrome.
Nature. 2015, 519 (7541), 92-96.

Slide 51 (Shown as 28):

Sujit S et al.
Polymers in the gut compress the colonic mucus hydrogel.
PNAS. 2016, June 28, 113 (26), 7041-7046; published ahead of print June 14.

Slide 52 (Shown as 29):

Tan M et al.
A pilot study on the percutaneous absorption of microfine titanium dioxide from sunscreens.
Australian Journal of Dermatology. 1996, 37 (4), 185-187

Waller T, Chen C & Walker SL.
Food and industrial grade titanium dioxide impacts gut microbiota.
Environmental Engineering Science. 2017, 34 (8), 537-550.

Heringa MB et al.
Detection of titanium particles in human liver and spleen and possible health implications.
Particle and Fibre Toxicology. 2018, 15 (1).

Brun E et al.
Titanium dioxide nanoparticle impact and translocation through ex vivo, in vivo and in vitro gut epithelia.
Particle and Fibre Toxicology. 2014, 11 (1), 13.

Slide 54 (Shown as 30):

Joly Condette et al.
Increased gut permeability and bacterial translocation after chronic Chlorpyrifos exposure in rats.
PloS ONE. 2014, 9 (7), e102217.

Slide 56 (Shown as 32):

Kish L et al.
Environmental particulate matter induces murine intestinal inflammatory responses and alters the gut microbiome.
PloS ONE. 2013, 8 (4), e62220.

Slide 59:

Viorica B et al.
Impact of oral Bisphenol A at reference doses on intestinal barrier function and sex differences after perinatal exposure in rats.
PNAS. 2010, January 5, 107 (1), 448-453.

DeLuca JA et al.
Bisphenol A alters microbiota metabolites derived from aromatic amino a-
cids and worsens disease activity during colitis.
Experimental Biology and Medicine. 2018, 243 (10), 864, 875.

Slide 60:

Yildiz HM et al.
Food-associated stimuli enhance barrier properties of gastrointestinal
mucus.
Biomaterials. 2015, 54, 1-8.

Slide 61:

Min-Hyun K.
The roles of glutamine in the intestine and its implication in intestinal dise-
ases.
Int J Mol Sci. 2017, May; 18 (5): 1051.

Basivireddy J et al.
Oral glutamine attenuates indomethacin-induced small intestinal damage.
Clinical Science. 2004, 107 (3), 281-289.

Slide 62 (Shown as 33):

Playford RJ et al.
Bovine colostrum is a health food supplement which prevents NSAID in-
duced gut damage.
Gut. 1999, 44 (5), 653-658.

Playford RJ et al.
Co-administration of the health food supplement, bovine colostrum, reduces the acute non-steroidal anti-inflammatory drug-induced increase in
intestinal permeability.
Clinical Science. 2001, 100 (6), 627.

Slide 63:

Ramadass B et al.
Sucrose co-administration reduces the toxic effect of lectin on gut permea-
bility and intestinal bacterial colonization.
Dis Sci. 2010, Oct; 55 (10): 2778-84.

Slide 64:

Stremmel W et al.
Delayed release phosphatidylcholine in chronic-active ulcerative colitis: a
randomized, double-blinded, dose-finding study.

J Clin Gastroenterol. 2010.

Stremmel W & Gauss A.
Lecithin as a therapeutic agent in ulcerative colitis.
Digestive Diseases. 2013, 31 (3-4), 388-390.

Slide 65:

Bischoff, SC et al.
Intestinal permeability - a new target for disease prevention and therapy.
BMC Gastroenterol. 2014, 14: 189.

Liu Z, Huang M et al.
Positive regulatory effects of perioperative probiotic treatment on postoperative liver complications after colorectal liver metastases surgery: a double-center and double-blind randomized clinical trial.
BMC Gastroenterol. 2015, 15: 34.

Orlando A et al.
Lactobacillus GG restoration of the gliadin induced epithelial barrier disruption: the role of cellular polyamines.
BMC Microbiol. 2014, 31; 14:19.

Slide 66:

Jianqin S et al.
Effects of milk containing only A2 beta casein versus milk containing both A1 and A2 beta casein proteins on gastrointestinal physiology, symptoms of discomfort, and cognitive behavior of people with self-reported intolerance to traditional cows' milk.
Nutr J. 2016, 15: 35.

Haupt-Jorgensen et al.
Possible prevention of diabetes with a gluten-free diet.
Nutrients. 2018, 10 (11), 1746.

Atkinson MA & Eisenbarth GS.
Type 1 diabetes: new perspectives on disease pathogenesis and treatment.
The Lancet. 2001, 358 (9277), 221-229.

Gorelick J et al.
The impact of diet wheat source on the onset of type 1 diabetes mellitus - Lessons learned from the non-obese diabetic (NOD) mouse model.
Nutrients. 2017, 9 (5), 482.

Slide 67 (Shown as 34):

Konijeti G et al.

Efficacy of the Autoimmune Protocol Diet for inflammatory bowel disease. *Inflammatory Bowel Diseases.* 2017, 23 (11), 2054-2060.

Sources Video 2

Slide 4 (Shown as 1):

Stefan A Müller-Lissner et al.
Myths and Misconceptions about chronic constipation.
American Journal of Gastroenterology. 2005. Blackwell Publishing.

Slide 5 (Shown as 2+3) :

Kok-Sun Ho et al.
Stopping or reducing dietary fiber intake reduces constipation and its associated symptoms.
World J Gastroenterol. 2012, September 7; 18 (33): 4593-4596.

Slide 10:

Alison MS & JH Cummings
Water-holding by dietary fibre in vitro and its relationship to faecal output in man.
Gut. 1979, 20, 722-729.

Slide 16 (Shown as 9):

Lawrence AD et al.
Diet rapidly and reproducibly alters the human gut microbiome.
Nature. 2014, Volume 505, 559-563.

Slide 17 (Shown as 10):

Chandalia M et al.
Beneficial effects of high dietary fiber intake in patients with type 2 diabetes mellitus.
New England Journal Medicine. 2000, 342: 1392-1398.

Slide 18 (Shown as 11):

Cannon MC & Frank Q.
Nuttall Diabetes.
American Diabetes Association. 2004, 53: 2375-2382.

Slide 22 (Shown as 5):

Triantafyllou K, Chang C & Pimentel M
Methanogens, methane and gastrointestinal Motility.
J Neurogastroenterol Motil. 2014, Jan; 20 (1): 31-40.
Slide 23:

Skodje GI et al.
Fructan, rather than gluten, induces symptoms in patients with self-reported non-celiac gluten sensitivity.
Gastroenterology. 2018 Feb; 154 (3): 529-539. e2.
https://www.gastrojournal.org/article/s0016-5085(17)36302-3/fulltext

Slide 25 (Shown as 15):

Mullin G et al.
Irritable Bowel Syndrome.
Journal of parenteral and enteral nutrition. 2014, 38, 10.
1177/0148607114545329.

Slide 29:

Ley RE et al.
Human gut microbes associated with obesity.
Nature. 2007, 444 (7122): 1022-3.

Slide 30 (Shown as 17):

Lawrence AD et al.
Diet rapidly and reproducibly alters the human gut microbiome.
Nature. 2014, Jan 23; 505 (7484): 559-63.

Slide 32:

Turnbaugh PJ et al.
An obesity-associated gut microbiome with increased capacity for energy harvest.
Nature. 2006, volume 444, page 1027-1031.

Slide 35 (Shown as 19):

Collins J et al.
Dietary trehalose enhances virulence of epidemic Clostridium Difficile.
Nature. 2018, V 553, 291-294.

Sources Video 3

Slide 6 (Shown as 5):

Sandoval M et al.
Pattern of weight loss after successful enucleation of an insulin-producing pancreatic neuroendocrine tumor.
Journal of the ASEAN Federation of Endocrine Societies. 2015, 30 (2), 159.

Slide 9 (Shown as 6):

Bao W et al.
Persistent elevation of plasma insulin levels is associated with increased cardiovascular risk in children and young adults. Heart Study.
Circulation. 1996, Jan 1; 93 (1); 54-9.

Slide 10 (Shown as 10+11+12):

Forster-Schubert KE et al.
Acyl and total ghrelin are suppressed strongly by ingested proteins, weakly by lipis, and biphasically by carbohydrates.
J Clin Endocrinol Metab. 2008 May, 93 (5): 1971-9.

Slide 14+15 (Shown as 8):

Ebbeling C et al.
Effects of a low carbohydrate diet on energy ependiture during weight loss maintenance: randomized trial.
BMJ. 2018 k4583.
https://elemental.medium.com/major-study-supports-carbohydrate-insulin-model-of-obesity-cb7d47a571d9

Slide 15:

Ebbeling CB et al.
Effects of dietary composition on energy expenditure during weight-loss maintenance.
JAMA. 2012, 307, 2627-34.

Slide 19 (Shown as 10):

Reaven G.
The metabolic syndrome or the insulin resistance syndromeDifferent names, different concepts, and different goals.
Endocrinol Metab Clin North Am. 2004, Jun; 33 (2); 283-303.

Smith U.

Impaired ('diabetic') insulin signaling and action occur in fat cells long before glucose intolerance-is insulin resistance initiated in the adipose tissue?
Int J Obes Relat Metab Disord. 2002; 26: 897-904.

Abbasi F et al.
The relationship between glucose disposal in response to physiological hyperinsulinemia and basal glucose and free fatty acid concentrations in healthy volunteers.
J Clin Endocrinol Metab. 2002, Mar; 85 (3): 1251-4

Slide 23+24 (Shown as 12+13):

Spalding KL et al.
Dynamics of fat cell turnover in humans.
Nature. 2008, 453 (7196): 783-7.

Slide 26 (Shown as 14):

Neeland IJ et al.
Visceral and ectoptic fat, atherosclerosis, and cardiometabolic disease: a position statement.
The Lancet Diabetes & Endocrinology. 2019 Sep; 7(9): 715-725.

Slide 27:

Gupta P et al.
The association between body composition using dual energy X-ray absorptiometry and type 2 diabetes: A systematic review and meta-analysis of observational studies.
Sci Rep. 2019, Sep 2; 9 (1): 12634.

Slide 28:

Meex RCR & Watt MJ et al.
Hepatokines: linking nonalcoholic fatty liver disease and insulin resistance.
Nature Reviews Endocrinology. 2017, 13 (9), 509-520.

Slide 31 (Shown as 15):

Peterson KF et al.
The role of skeletal muscle insulin resistance in the pathogenesis of the metabolic syndrome.
NAS. 2007, July 31, 104 (31), 12587-12594.

Slide 33 (see 8):

Slide 34:

Waninge A et al.
Measuring waist circumference in disabled adults.
Research in Developmental Disabilities. 2010, 31 (3), 839-847.

Slide 36:

Gonzales-Saldivar et al.
Skin manifestations of insulin resistance: From a biochemical stance to a linical diagnosis and management.
Dermatol Ther (Heidelb). 2017, Mar; 7(1): 37-51.

Slide 44 (Shown as 22):

Athinarayanan SJ et al.
Long-term effects of a novel continuous remote care intervention including nutritional ketosis for the management of type 2 diabetes: A 2-year non-randomized clinical trial.
Frontiers in Endocrinology. 2019, 10.

Slide 47 (Shown as 24):

Ceriello A et al.
Oscillating glucose is more deleterious to endothelial function and oxidative stress than mean glucose in normal and type 2 diabetic patients.
Diabetes. 2008, 57: 1349-1354.

Slide 48:

Srour B et al.
Ultra-processed food intake and risk of cardiovascular disease: prospective cohort study. (NutriNet-Sante)
BMJ. l1451.

Monteiro CA et al.
Ultra-processed foods: what they are and how to identify them.
Public Health Nutrition. 2019, 1-6.

Slide 58 (Shown as 28):

Hyde PN et al.
Dietary carbohydrate restriction improves metabolic syndrome independant of weight loss.
JCI Insight. 2019, 4 (12).
Slide 60 (Shown as 30):

Ramirez MR et al.

Effect of the type of frying culinary fat on volatile compounds isolated in fried pork loin chops by using SPME-GC-MS.
Journal of Agricultural and Food Chemistry. 2004, 52 (25), 7637-7643.

Slide 61 (Shown as 31):

Mu H et al.
Study on the volatile oxidation compounds and quantitave prediction of oxidation parameters in walnut (Carya cathayensis Sarg.) oil.
European Journal of Lipid Science and Technology. 2019, 1800521.

Slide 63 (Shown as 32):

Staprans I et al.
The role of dietary oxidized cholesterol and oxidized fatty acids in the development of atherosclerosis.
Molecular Nutrition & Food Research. 2005, 49 (11), 1075-1082.

Slide 64:

Bieghs V et al.
Trapping of oxidized LDL in lysosomes of Kupffer cells is a trigger for hepatic inflammation.
Liver International. 2013, 33 (7), 1056-1061.

Slide 65:

Ho CM et al.
Accumulation of free cholesterol and oxidized low-density lipoprotein is associated with portal inflammation and fibrosis in nonalcoholic fatty liver disease.
Journal of Inflammation. 2019, 16 (1).

Slide 66 (Shown as 33):

Cavicchi M et al.
Prevalence of liver disease and contributing factors in patients recovering home parenteral nutrition for permanent intestinal failure.
Annals of Internal Medicine. 2000, 132 (7), 525.

Slide 68 (Shown as 35):

Staprans I et al.
The role of dietary oxidized cholesterol and oxidized fatty acids in the development of atherosclerosis.
Molecular Nutrition & Food Research. 2005, 49 (11), 1075-1082.

Slide 70 (Shown as 36):

Dehghan M et al.
Associations of fats and carbohydrate intake with cardiovascular disease and mortality in 18 countries from five continents (PURE): a prospective cohort study.
Lancet. 2017, Nov 4; 390 (10107): 2050-2062.

Slide 72 (Shown as 37):

Ravnskov U et al.
Lack of an association or an inverse association between low-density-lipoprotein cholesterol and mortaliy in the elderly: a systematic review.
BMJ Open. 2016, 6: e010401.

Other Revised Transcripts Publications

The carnivore diet of Dr. Jordan Peterson and Mikhaila Peterson
How meat healed their depression, anxiety and diseases
Revised Transcripts and Blogposts. Featuring Dr. Shawn Baker

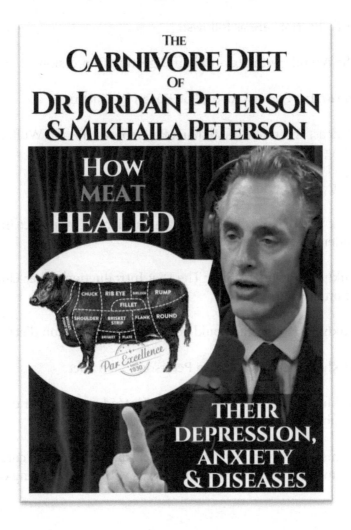

This book offers 11 Chapters of revised transcripts of Dr. Jordan Peterson & Mikhaila Peterson on:

- how they cured their disease, depression and health issues with the carnivore diet and

- how ill people could start this kind of eating as well.

The Transcripts are as follows:

1. The Agenda with Steve Paikin Digesting Depression

2. Joe Rogan Podcast 1070 3. Joe Rogan Podcast 1139

4. Podcast Interview of Mikhaila Peterson with Robb Wolf, including blood work

5. Podcast Interview with Ivor Cummins

6. Talk by Mikhaila Peterson at the Carnivore Conference in Boulder, 2019

7. Mikhaila Petersons Blog: The Diet Introduction of her Lion Diet on YouTube

8. Mikhaila Peterson: Should you start an elimination diet?

9. Mikhaila Peterson: Jordan Peterson's Lion Diet

10 Mikhaila Peterson: The Lion Diet (Introduction of her diet on YouTube

11. Bonus-Transcript: Dr. Shawn Baker talking about his coronary calcium score and overall health status with years of being carnivore.

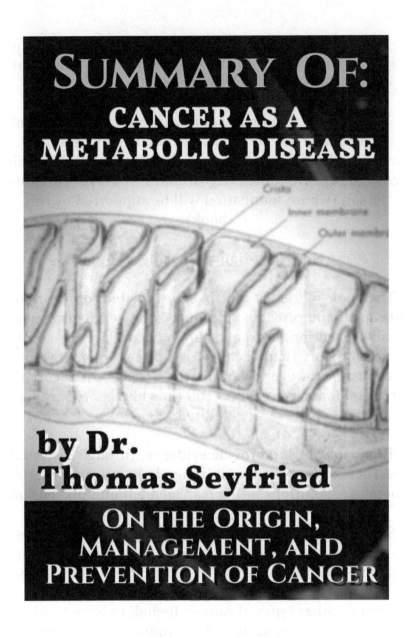

25% of the royalties of this book will be donated to Dr. Seyfrieds research!
See www.KetoforCancer.net for our current donation status!

This research will actually make a REAL impact, as it studies the real causes and treatment opportunities of cancer!

This book is a summary of Dr. Thomas Seyfrieds book "Cancer as a metabolic disease" and comprises transcripts of his talks and interviews, as well as texts by his collegue Dr. Dominic D'Agostiono and Travis Christofferson (whose foundation will be supported by this book).

Here the original Book description:

The book addresses controversies related to the origins of cancer and provides solutions to cancer management and prevention. It expands upon Otto Warburg's well-known theory that all cancer is a disease of energy metabolism. However, Warburg did not link his theory to the "hallmarks of cancer" and thus his theory was discredited.

This book aims to provide evidence, through case studies, that cancer is primarily a metabolic disease requring metabolic solutions for its management and prevention.

Support for this position is derived from critical assessment of current cancer theories. Brain cancer case studies are presented as a proof of principle for metabolic solutions to disease management, but similarities are drawn to other types of cancer, including breast and colon, due to the same cellular mutations that they demonstrate.

SUMMARY OF:

The
Obesity Code

&

The
Diabetes Code

by Dr.
Jason Fung

UNLOCKING THE SECRETS OF WEIGHT LOSS / REVERSE TYPE 2 DIABETES

25% of the royalties of this book will be donated to Dr. Fungs research and work!

This book is a summary of Dr. Jason Fung's books "The Obesity Code" and "The Diabetes Code" by revising Dr. Fungs own transcripts.

<u>Here the original Book description of "The Obesity Code":</u>

The landmark book from New York Times-bestselling author Dr. Jason Fung, one of the world's leading experts on intermittent fasting for weight-loss and longevity, whose 5-step plan has helped thousands of people lose weight and achieve lasting health.

Everything you believe about how to lose weight is wrong. Weight gain and obesity are driven by hormones—in everyone—and only by understanding the effects of insulin and insulin resistance can we achieve lasting weight loss.

In this highly readable and provocative book, Dr. Jason Fung sets out an original, robust theory of obesity that provides startling insights into proper nutrition.

In addition to his five basic steps, a set of lifelong habits that will improve your health and control your insulin levels, Dr. Fung explains how to use intermittent fasting to break the cycle of insulin resistance and reach a healthy weight—for good.

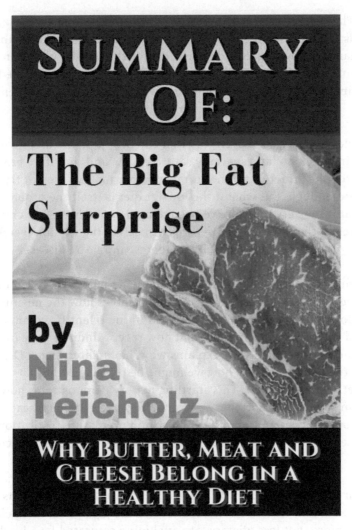

SUMMARY OF:

The Big Fat Surprise

by Nina Teicholz

WHY BUTTER, MEAT AND CHEESE BELONG IN A HEALTHY DIET

25% of the royalties of this book will be donated to Mrs. Teicholz' foundation The Nutrition Coaltion (which works towards an evidence based decision making process regarding the US Dietary Guidelines)

This book is a summary of Nina Teicholz' book "The Obesity Code" and "The Diabetes Code" by revising her own transcripts.

Here the original Book description:

In The Big Fat Surprise, investigative journalist Nina Teicholz reveals the unthinkable: that everything we thought we knew about dietary fat is wrong. She documents how the low-fat nutrition advice of the past sixty years has amounted to a vast uncontrolled experiment on the entire population, with disastrous consequences for our health.

For decades, we have been told that the best possible diet involves cutting back on fat, especially saturated fat, and that if we are not getting healthier or thinner it must be because we are not trying hard enough. But what if the low-fat diet is itself the problem? What if the very foods we've been denying ourselves—the creamy cheeses, the sizzling steaks—are themselves the key to reversing the epidemics of obesity, diabetes, and heart disease?

In this captivating, vibrant, and convincing narrative, based on a nine-year-long investigation, Teicholz shows how the misinformation about saturated fats took hold in the scientific community and the public imagination, and how recent findings have overturned these beliefs. She explains why the Mediterranean Diet is not the healthiest, and how we might be replacing trans fats with something even worse. This startling history demonstrates how nutrition science has gotten it so wrong: how overzealous researchers, through a combination of ego, bias, and premature institutional consensus, have allowed dangerous misrepresentations to become dietary dogma.

With eye-opening scientific rigor, The Big Fat Surprise upends the conventional wisdom about all fats with the groundbreaking claim that more, not less, dietary fat—including saturated fat—is what leads to better health and wellness. Science shows that we have been needlessly avoiding meat, cheese, whole milk, and eggs for decades and that we can now, guilt-free, welcome these delicious foods back into our lives.

Sources

CHAPTER:

1) Text basis for the transcriptions, Images, Graphics::
Video on YouTube:

Channel: see above

Titel: Dr. Paul Mason - 'Evidence based keto: How to lose weight and reverse diabetes'

Video-Url: https://www.youtube.com/watch?v=xqUO4P9ADIo

2) Text basis for the transcription:

Channel: Low Carb Down Under

Channel-Url: see above

Titel: Dr. Paul Mason - 'From fibre to the

microbiome: low carb gut health'

Video-Url: https://www.youtube.com/watch?v=xqUO4P9ADIo

3) Text basis for the transcription:

Channel: Low Carb Down Under

Channel-Url: https://www.youtube.com/channel/UCcTTiHZtNpiqD2EubIO5HFw

Title: Dr. Paul Mason - 'How lectins impact your health - from obesity to autoimmune disease'

Video-Url: https://www.youtube.com/watch?v=mjQZCCiV6iA